Sirtfoo Diet Cookbook

How to Lose Weight, Activate Your Metabolism, Eat Healthy with Carnivorous, Vegan, and Vegetarian Recipes

APRIL DANIELLE FLORES

INTRODUCTION

Congratulations on purchasing *Sirtfood Diet Cookbook*, and thank you for doing so. The food options on the Sirtfood Diet will provide you with health benefits, including anti-inflammatory and antioxidant properties.

The Sirtfood Diet is restrictive concerning foods and calories, which makes it challenging to remain on for extended times. The goal of the diet is to help people lose weight quickly, eat healthily, and feel energized. You will want to do a sufficient amount of exercise to have more success with your diet plan.

You should also chat with your physician before you begin dieting to ensure your body is ready for changes that are used with lifestyle change. However, if you have heard and thought "the idea of switching on your skinny gene," it isn't supported by extensive research at this time.

This guideline will help you realize whether the Sirtfood Diet is for you or not. First, here is a bit of history for the Sirtfood Diet.

The U.K. was the first to publish a book for the diet plan in 2016. A pair of authors and health consultants, Aidan Goggins and Glen Matten were focused on healthy eating rather than weight loss. The research evolved into a diet rich in powerful "sirtuin-activating-polyphenols," resulting in wonder foods called "Sirtfoods."

Originators of the Sirtfood Diet claim, if you eat specific foods, they will trigger your "skinny gene" pathway. Thus providing you with the ability to lose "seven pounds in seven days." The plan includes polyphenols which are natural chemicals including foods such as wine, dark chocolate, and kale. You should also incorporate turmeric, cinnamon, and red onions. These are the foods that will jump-start the 'sirtuin pathway' to initiate weight loss.

The plan was outlined as follows:

Phase 1: Initiation Phase is For Seven Days

During the initial phase, you may experience side effects, including irritability, fatigue, or lightheadedness. Unfortunately, most plans that lower caloric intake can cause issues. In the first three days, you will be allowed one meal and three sirtfood green juices totaling 1,000 calories. For days four to seven, you can enjoy two meals and two green juices, equalling 1,500 calories.

Phase 2: 14-Day Maintenance Plan

This phase is not designed to maintain your current weight. Its purpose is to allow you to lose weight steadily. You will have three balanced meals and one green juice daily.

According to *Healthline*, the diet will help you drop the pounds since it's low in calories. However, the weight possibly will return at the end of the diet plan. Since the diet isn't long-term, it should not have any adverse effects on your health.

I have provided you with a strict diet plan for four weeks. The fourth week is a plan where you can enjoy eating the sirtfood foods - your own way. The last chapters will include a variety of food options to choose from if there is an item on the meal plan that just isn't your favorite.

Chapter 1: The Sirtfood Diet Foundation

Know Whether the Diet Is For You

It is vital to discuss the diet with your doctor. Factors including, your sex, age, BMI, current medications, and lifestyle. All play a part in your favor for the diet. It may not be for you. Don't try the Sirtfood Diet if you have any of the following:

- A complicated medical history.
- A BMI of less than 30.
- You suffer from IBD/IBS.
- You have hypoglycemia.
- You are on antidepressants.
- You are on other medications.
- If you are allergic to most foods mentioned on the Sirtfood's list.

Learn How Exercise Fits into The Diet Plan

It's time for you to decide whether the Sirtfood techniques are a way of life rather than a "fad" diet. If you have tried other plans and found it too challenging to drop the pounds, the Sirtfood plan can help with that struggle.

But remember, it is advised to enjoy yourself and eat foods that can generate your "skinny gene" pathways, which can be activated by exercise and fasting processes. You will be on target because foods, including red wine and chocolate, contain polyphenols, which will enable the genes to mimic the effects of exercising and fasting.

According to the Sirtfood pros, during the first couple of weeks, while the calories are reduced, listen to your body. Do not work out if you have lowered energy or feel fatigued. Stay focused on a healthier lifestyle, including your daily levels of fruits, veggies, and fiber.

After you have adjusted your lifestyle, be sure you consume protein before a workout. It's valuable to repair your muscles and reduce the soreness to aid recovery after exercise. For example, drink a Sirt Blueberry Smoothie (enclosed in the recipe section) if you would like a light boost. You could also have a bowl of Sirt Chili Con Carne or one of the many other options provided in your new cookbook.

Possible Side Effects

When you first begin the diet, the green juice may cause you to feel nauseous, impair your mental focus, or have a headache. You may have bad breath which is a possible side effect from not eating enough food. Digestive complications may also be an issue if you are not consuming enough fiber. You may be cranky or hungry since the calories are probably much lower than you currently use.

After you use the following meal plan for the four weeks included, you will have a better understanding of how to lose weight whenever you choose. I have provided you with the guidelines, followed by the type of meal/juice and the calories for that item. If there is food for the day you do not like, look through the index and discover an alternative with the same amount of calories. It's that easy, so let's get juicing and cooking!

Know The Sirtfood Menu Items

Apples: You already know apples are delicious, but they are also low in cholesterol, fat, and sodium with excellent sources for fiber and Vitamin C. For just 100 calories, indulge in one medium-sized apple for a quick snack.

Citrus Fruits: Citrus fruits are also abundant in multiple other nutrients, including potassium calcium, folate, niacin, thiamin, vitamin B6, magnesium, phosphorus, riboflavin, copper, and pantothenic acid.

Red Wine: On average, a glass of red wine will give you 1 % of vitamin K,

3 % riboflavin (or vitamin B2), 1 % thiamin, 2 % niacin, 2 % choline, and trace amounts of other essential minerals.

Buckwheat: Reduce your blood sugar, improve heart health, and protect against cancer. It is also gluten-free and rich in dietary fiber.

Walnuts: The nuts are a super plant source of omega-3s and rich in antioxidants. It may also decrease inflammation and promote a healthy gut. It supports weight control and may also help manage type 2 diabetes and lower blood pressure.

Dark Chocolate: Use dark chocolate for your baking needs because it is one of the best antioxidants on the planet (according to studies). It can also lower your risk of heart disease and improve your health.

Medjool Dates: The dates are high in calories, but full of nutrients and antioxidants that are linked to many health benefits. In particular, their fiber may boost digestion and heart health while lowering your risk of several chronic diseases.

Parsley: Enjoy the benefits of parsley as an important part of the plan with its healthy nutrients to support bone health. It is also rich in antioxidants, cancer-fighting substances, can improve your heart health, and has antibacterial properties.

Capers: Add capers to your diet plan to supply natural antioxidants. Capers are showing promising effects for those who suffer from heart disease or for those who are fighting cancer.

Blueberries: The berries are an antioxidant superfood packed with phytoflavinoids, and high in Vitamin C and potassium, making them one of the top choices of doctors and nutritionists. The berries can lower the risk of cancer and heart disease.

Green Tea: Enjoy green tea to improve blood flow, lower cholesterol and help prevent blood pressure issues and heart failure.

Soy: Soy is high in protein, fiber, cholesterol-free, and lactose-free. It is also an excellent source of antioxidants, omega-3fatty acids, and high in phytoestrogens.

Strawberries: The berries are packed with fiber, vitamins, and particularly high levels of antioxidants. Strawberries are a fat-free, low-calorie, sodium-free, cholesterol-free food. They are also an excellent source of potassium and manganese.

Turmeric: The spice turmeric's most active compound is curcumin that has many scientifically-proven health benefits, such as the potential to prevent cancer, heart disease, Alzheimer's, depression, and arthritis pain.

Olive Oil: Olive oil protects against inflammation. It helps reduce oxidation of LDL (bad) cholesterol, improves blood vessel health, helps lower your blood pressure, and also helps manage blood clotting.

Red Onion: Most of the benefits come from antioxidants. Research shows that one particular antioxidant, called quercetin, protects health in several ways. One study shows that quercetin fights inflammation and boosts the immune system. Research mainly conducted in labs has shown that onions may kill a wide range of bacteria.

Garden Rocket - Arugula: The benefits include calcium which can help the blood to normally clot and potassium that is vital for nerve and heart function. It is also loaded with Folate (B Vitamin), Vitamin C, and Vitamin K which also assists with blood coagulation.

Kale: Many health benefits are derived from one of the most nutrient-dense foods on the planet, including its powerful antioxidants, vitamin C and Vitamin K.

Delicious Prepared Snacks

Blackberries
Servings: 1
Nutritional Calories: 32
Ingredients Needed:

- Blackberries (15)

1. All you need to do for this delicious treat is to rinse the berries.
2. Pop them into the fridge to chill or freeze them for another time.

Blueberries
Servings: 1
Nutritional Calories: 36

1. Grab a large handful and enjoy them anytime you need a boost.

Olives
Servings: 1
Nutritional Calories: 75
Ingredients Needed:

- Olives (6 large)

1. Serve a platter of delicious olives as an appetizer or snack. Serve them unchilled for a fuller flavor.

Pomegranate Seeds
Servings: 1
Nutritional Calories: 50
Ingredients Needed:

- Seeds (half of 1 small pkg./50g)

This fabulous on-the-go snack is excellent for your dieting method.

Red Apples
Servings: 1
Nutritional Calories: 47

Always have one or two in the fridge for a quick pick-up anytime.

Red Grapes
Servings: 10 grapes
Nutritional Calories: 30

Store a bunch of grapes in the fridge for a quick and easy snack.

Chapter 2: Phase 1 Day 1-3

Day one through three, you will have the same green juice. You will enjoy one meal with three green juices. You will also have a 1000 calorie limit.

Day 1: Daily Total: 919 Calories

Juice 1: Sirtfood Green Juice: 120
Time Required: 10-15 minutes
Servings: 2
Nutritional Calories: 120

Ingredients Needed:

- Arugula/rocket (30g/1 large handful)
- Kale (75g/2 large handfuls)
- Flat-leaf parsley (5g/1 small handful)
- Celery (150g - including leaves/2-3 large stalks)
- Optional: Lovage leaves (5g/1 small handful)
- Lemon juice (half of 1 lemon)
- Green apple (half of 1 medium)
- Matcha green tea (.5 level tsp.)

Method for Preparation:

1. Mix the greens (parsley, rocket, lovage, and kale) and juice them. (You want about 50ml/.21 cup of juice.)
2. Juice the apple and celery. Peel the lemon by hand (not a knife). You should have about one cup of juice or maybe more.
3. Add the tea when it's time to serve. Pour a small portion into a serving

glass and mix in the matcha. After the matcha has dissolved, combine it with the rest of the juice.
4. Pour it into two glasses and serve immediately.
5. Take care to use this drink for the first two drinks in the diet plan, since it contains caffeine, and shouldn't be consumed late in the day.
6. Note: * Fresh lovage leaves have a yeast-like, sharp, and musky taste with a lemony-celery-like aroma. Dried leaves have a more robust flavor.

Juice 2: Green Fruit Juice - No Kale: 304

Time Required: 10 minutes
Servings: 2
Nutritional Calories: 304

Ingredients Needed:

- Kiwi (3 large)
- Fresh lime juice (2 tsp.)
- Green apples (3 large)
- Seedless green grapes (2 cups)

Method for Preparation:

1. Peel and chop the kiwi. Slice and core the apples.
2. Toss each of the ingredients into a juicer.
3. Remove the juice and pour it into two glasses to serve.

Juice 3: Celery Juice: 32

Time Required: 10 minutes
Servings: 2
Nutritional Calories: 32

Ingredients Needed:

- Celery stalks with leaves (8)
- Fresh ginger (2 tbsp.)
- Lemon (1)
- Filtered water (.5 cup)
- Salt (1 pinch)

Method for Preparation:

1. Peel the lemon and ginger.
2. Toss each of the fixings into a blender and thoroughly puree until incorporated.
3. Strain the juice using a mesh strainer.
4. Serve in two glasses right away.

Meal for the Day: Chicken & Veggies with Buckwheat Noodles 463

Time Required: 45 minutes
Servings: 2
Nutritional Calories: 463

Ingredients Needed:

- Broccoli florets (.5 cup)
- Fresh green beans (.5 cup)
- Buckwheat noodles (5 oz.)
- Fresh kale (1 cup)
- Coconut oil (1 tbsp.)
- Brown onion (1)
- Cubed chicken breast (6 oz.)
- Garlic (2 cloves)
- Soy sauce - low-sodium (3 tbsp.)

Method for Preparation:

1. Trim and slice the beans. Remove the tough kale ribs and chop them. Finely chop the cloves and onion. Cube the chicken.
2. Prepare a pan of boiling water. Toss in the green beans and broccoli to steam for four to five minutes.
3. Toss in the kale, and cook another one to two minutes.
4. Drain the veggies and place them in a container. Set them aside for now.
5. Prepare another pan with boiling salted water and cook the noodles for five minutes.
6. Drain and rinse the noodles.
7. Prepare a large wok with oil. Using medium heat, toss in and sauté the onion for two to three minutes. Fold in the cubed chicken and cook for another five to six minutes.
8. Mix in the soy sauce, garlic, and a splash of water. Simmer for two to three minutes, stirring often.
9. Stir in the veggies and noodles. Warm everything for one to two minutes, before serving with a garnish of sesame seeds.

Day 2: Daily Total: 880 Calories

Juice 1: Sirtfood Green Juice: 120
Enjoy the same juice used for day 1.

Juice 2: Apple & Cucumber Juice: 230
Time Required: 10-12 minutes
Servings: 2
Nutritional Calories: 230

Ingredients Needed:

- Large apples (3)
- Cucumbers (2 large)
- Celery (4 stalks)
- Fresh ginger (1-inch/2.5cm piece)
- Lemon (1)

Method for Preparation:

1. Core and slice the apples and cucumbers. Peel the lemon and ginger.
2. Add each of the fixings into a juicer and extract the juice according to the manufacturer's directions.
3. Pour it into two chilled glasses to serve immediately.

Juice 3: Kale - Carrot & Grapefruit Juice: 232
Time Required: 10 minutes
Servings: 2
Nutritional Calories: 232

Ingredients Needed:

- Granny Smith apple (2 large)
- Fresh kale (3 cups)
- Fresh juice (1 tsp./1 lemon)
- Grapefruit (2 medium)
- Carrots (2)

Method for Preparation:

1. Peel the carrots and grapefruit. Slice and core the apple. Chop the carrots. Section the grapefruit, and squeeze the juice.
2. Toss the prepared foods into the juicer.

3. Extract the juice and pour it into two cold glasses to serve.

Meal for the Day: Shrimp with Broccoli & Carrots: 298
Time Required: 23-25 minutes
Servings: 5
Nutritional Calories: 298

Ingredients Needed:
The Sauce:

- Fresh ginger (1 tbsp.)
- Garlic (2 cloves)
- Red wine vinegar (1 tbsp.)
- Soy sauce - l.s. (3 tbsp.)
- Red pepper flakes (.25 tsp.)
- Brown sugar (1 tsp.)

The Shrimp Mixture:

- Olive oil (3 tbsp.)
- Medium shrimp (1.5 lb.)
- Broccoli florets (12 oz.)
- Carrots (8 oz.)

Method for Preparation:

1. Peel and devein the shrimp. Grate the ginger and mince the garlic. Peel and slice the carrots.
2. Toss all of the sauce fixings in a bowl and whisk until combined.
3. Prep a large wok using the med-high temperature setting and heat the oil.
4. Toss in the shrimp to sauté for about two minutes, tossing intermittently.
5. Toss in the carrots and broccoli. Sauté them for three to four minutes, stirring often.
6. Mix in the sauce and simmer for one to two minutes and serve.

Day 3: Daily Total: 915 Calories

Juice 1: Sirtfood Green Juice: 120
Serve yourself another green juice.

Juice 2: Apple-Celery Juice: 240
Time Required: 10 minutes
Servings: 2

Nutritional Calories: 240

Ingredients Needed:

- Green apples (4 large)
- Celery stalks (4)
- Lemon (1)

Method for Preparation:

1. Peel, core, and slice the apples. Peel the lemon.
2. Toss the fixings into a juicer.
3. When it's ready, pour into two glasses and serve.

Juice 3: Broccoli - Apple & Orange Juice: 254

Time Required: 10 minutes
Servings: 2
Nutritional Calories: 254

Ingredients Needed:

- Broccoli (2 stalks)
- Sliced green apples (2 large)
- Oranges (3 large)
- Fresh parsley (4 tbsp.)

Method for Preparation:

1. Core the apples and chop the broccoli. Peel and section the oranges.
2. Toss all of the components into a juicer and extract the juice.
3. Pour and serve in two glasses to serve right away for the best flavor.

Meal for the Day: Grilled Lamb Chops & Kale: 301

Time Required: 26-30 minutes
Servings: 4
Nutritional Calories: 301

Ingredients Needed:

- Garlic (1 clove)
- Fresh rosemary leaves (1 tbsp.)
- Loin chops (4)

- Fresh baby kale (4 cups)
- Salt and black pepper (as desired)

Method for Preparation:

1. Mince the garlic and rosemary.
2. Warm the grill using the high-temperature setting and lightly grease the grill grate.
3. Whisk the salt, pepper, rosemary, and garlic in a mixing bowl. Cover the chops with the mixture. Arrange them on the grill to cook for approximately two minutes per side.
4. Arrange the chops to the cooler side of the grill and simmer another six to seven minutes.
5. Portion the kale on the plates and top each one with a chop to serve.

Chapter 3: Phase 1 Day 4-7

You are still in phase one of the Sirtfood Diet plan, but the calories are increased to 1500 daily. You will have two green juice options and two meals during these days. However, you will drink the same Sirtfood Green Juice with 120 calories for the entirety of Phase One.

Day 4: 1536 Calories

Green Juice 1: Sirtfood Green Juice: 120
Enjoy the same green juice used for day 1.

Green Juice 2: Lemony Green Juice: 196
Time Required: 10 minutes
Servings: 2
Nutritional Calories: 196

Ingredients Needed:
- Green apples (2 large)
- Fresh kale leaves (4 cups/67g)
- Fresh parsley leaves (4 tbsp./3.8g)
- Fresh ginger (1-inch piece/2.5cm/1 tbsp.)
- Lemon (1)
- Filtered water (.5 cup/4 oz.)
- Salt (1 pinch)

Method for Preparation:

1. Remove the core and slice the apples. Peel the lemon and ginger.
2. Toss the fixings into a blender and mix until incorporated.
3. Remove and work it through a fine-mesh strainer to remove the juice.
4. Empty the juice into two chilled glasses and serve.

Meal 1: Miso-Marinated Baked Cod & Greens: 355

Time Required: 1 hour 10 minutes
Servings: 1
Nutritional Calories: 355

Ingredients Needed:

- Olive oil (1 tbsp.)
- Mirin (1 tbsp.)
- Miso (20g/.75 oz./3.5 tsp.)
- Cod fillet - skinless (1.7 oz./200g)
- Red onion (⅛ cup/.75 oz./20g)
- Celery (⅜ cup/40g/1.5 oz.)
- Garlic cloves (2)
- Thai chili - bird's eye (1)
- Fresh ginger (1 tsp.)
- Green beans (⅜ cup/60g/2 oz.)
- Kale (1 ⅝ oz./.75 cup/50g)
- Sesame seeds (1 tsp.)
- Parsley (5g/2 tbsp.)
- Tamari/soy sauce (1 tbsp.)
- Buckwheat (.25 cup/42.5g)
- Ground turmeric (1 tsp.)

Method for Preparation:

1. Slice the celery and onion. Mince the garlic, ginger, and chili. Roughly chop the parsley and kale.
2. Whisk the mirin, miso, and one teaspoon of oil. Rub it over the fish. Set it aside to marinate it for about half an hour.
3. Warm the oven to reach 425° Fahrenheit/ 220°Celsius
4. Set the timer and bake the cod for ten minutes.
5. Warm a skillet/wok and heat the remaining oil. Toss in the onion to stir fry for two to three minutes. Toss in the garlic, celery, green beans, kale, and chili. Stir-fry or toss until the kale is fork-tender, adding water as needed.
6. Prepare the buckwheat according to the package directions and toss

with the turmeric. Mix in the tamari, parsley, and sesame seeds to serve.

Meal 1: Side Dish: Kale & Citrus Fruit Salad: 256

Time Required: 15 minutes
Servings: 2
Nutritional Calories: 256

Ingredients Needed:

- Fresh kale (3 cups)
- Orange (1)
- Grapefruit (1)
- Dried cranberries (2 tbsp. - unsweetened)
- White sesame seeds (.25 tsp.)

The Dressing:

- Dijon mustard (1 tsp.)
- Raw honey (.5 tsp.)
- Olive oil (2 tbsp.)
- Orange juice (2 tbsp.)
- Pepper and salt (as desired)

Method for Preparation:

1. Trim away the ribs from the kale and tear them apart.
2. Peel the orange and grapefruit. Break them into segments.
3. Toss everything for the salad into two bowls.
4. Prepare the dressing components and shake well in a salad mixing jar.
5. Serve each salad with a portion of dressing.

Meal 2: Chickpea - Quinoa & Turmeric Curry: 609

Time Required: 1 hour 20 minutes
Servings: 6
Nutritional Calories: 609

Ingredients Needed:

- New potatoes (500g)
- Garlic (3 cloves)
- Ground ginger (1 tsp.)
- Turmeric (3 tsp.)

- Chili flakes (1 tsp.)
- Ground coriander (1 tsp.)
- Coconut milk (200 ml)
- Crushed tomatoes (400g can)
- Quinoa (180g)
- Boiling water (300 ml)
- Chickpeas (400g can)
- Spinach (150g)
- Pepper and salt (to your liking)

Method for Preparation:

1. Drain and rinse the chickpeas. Toss the potatoes into a pot of cold water and wait for it to boil. Cook them for 25 minutes until they are easily sliced into halves (drain and slice).
2. Pour the potatoes, tomatoes, milk, ginger, chili, coriander, turmeric, and garlic into a large pan and simmer until they begin boiling. Add in the quinoa.
3. Lower the temperature setting, put a top on the pot, and simmer it for about 45 minutes. Slowly add a mug of boiling water, stirring every 15 minutes (or so).
4. Halfway through, add the chickpeas.
5. Once the quinoa has cooked and is fluffy, not crunchy, it's ready. Stir through most of the spinach and seasonings as desired.
6. Serve using a handful of spinach leaves to garnish.

Day 5: 1427 Calories

Green Juice 1: Sirtfood Green Juice: 120
Enjoy your morning after your glass of juice!

Green Juice 2: Grape & Melon Juice: 125
Time Required: 2-3 minutes
Servings: 1
Nutritional Calories: 125

Ingredients Needed:

- Cucumber (half of 1)
- Spinach (30g baby leaves)

- Green grapes (100g)
- Cantaloupe melon (100g)

Method for Preparation:

1. Peel and deseed the melon of choice into chunks.
2. Peel (or not) the cucumber, remove the seeds and chop it. Remove the stalks from the spinach.
3. Combine all of the fixings in a juicer or blender. Work the mixture until it's creamy smooth.

Meal 1: Pancakes With Blackcurrants & Apples: 470

Time Required: 50-55 minutes
Servings: 4
Nutritional Calories: 470

Ingredients Needed:

- Apples (2)
- Baking powder (1 tsp.)
- Quick-cooking oats (2 cups)
- Raw sugar/coconut sugar/warm honey (2 tbsp.)
- Flour (1 cup)
- Egg whites (2)
- Milk - soy/coconut/rice (1.25 cups)
- Olive oil (2 tsp.)
- Salt (1 dash)

The Topping:

- Blackcurrants (1 cup)
- Sugar (2 tbsp.)
- Water (3 tbsp. or less)

Method for Preparation:

1. Peel and slice the apples into small chunks. Rinse and remove the stalks from the blackcurrants.
2. Simmer the topping ingredients in a saucepan for about ten minutes, stirring often.
3. Whisk the dry fixings and add the apples. Mix and add the milk slowly to make the batter.
4. Whisk the whites of egg and mix them in. Place the mix in the fridge.
5. Add ¼ of the oil into a skillet and add the batter. When done, serve with the berries.

Meal 2: Coq Au Vin: 459

Time Required: 45 minutes
Servings: 4
Nutritional Calories: 459

Ingredients Needed:

- Olive oil (1 tbsp.)
- Red onion (1)
- Chicken thighs (600g)
- French red wine - ex. Cotes du Rhone (.75 cup)
- Chicken stock/Bouillon cube is okay (.75 cup)
- Bay leaves (2)
- Thyme (2 sprigs)
- Pepper & Salt (to taste)
- Smoked bacon/lardons (3 oz.)
- Chestnut mushrooms (3.5 oz.)

To Serve:

- Green vegetables
- New potatoes (14 oz.)

Method for Preparation:

1. Chop the onion, bacon, and mushrooms. Remove any bones and skin from the chicken. Warm a saucepan with the oil. Toss in the onions and sauté them using the med-low temperature setting until softened (3 min.),
2. Adjust the temperature to medium to cook the chicken fillets (3 min.). Stir intermittently until they are slightly browned.
3. Pour in the stock, wine, thyme, and bay leaves. After it's boiling, adjust the temperature setting to a low setting and let it simmer. Put a lid on the pot.
4. Warm a cast-iron skillet using high heat for one minute, and add the bacon to cook for one minute. Fold in the mushrooms to sauté for another two minutes until they're browned. Toss them into the stew. Put the lid on the pot and simmer it for another 15 minutes. Remove the lid, stir and simmer with the lid off.
5. While the stew is simmering, steam the potatoes for 15 minutes and a green veggie for five minutes or until softened.
6. Serve the Coq au Vin with the veggies, new potatoes, and a delicious glass of wine.

Meal 2: Side Dish: Kale - Apple & Cranberry Salad: 253
Time Required: 15 minutes
Servings: 4
Nutritional Calories: 253

Ingredients Needed:
- Baby kale (6 cups)
- Apples (3 large - cored & sliced)
- Sliced almonds (.25 cup)
- Dried cranberries (.25 cup unsweetened)
- Raw honey (1 tbsp.)
- Olive oil (2 tbsp.)
- Salt and black pepper (as desired)

Method for Preparation:
1. Toss each of the fixings into a fancy salad bowl.
2. Mix well and serve to enjoy them promptly for the best flavor results.

Day 6: 1528 Calories

Green Juice 1: Sirtfood Green Juice: 120
Have another tasty Sirtfood juice this morning.

Green Juice 2: Kale & Fruit Juice: 293
Time Required: 10 minutes
Servings: 2
Nutritional Calories: 293

Ingredients Needed:
- Green apples (2 large)
- Fresh kale (3 cups)
- Large pears (2)
- Celery (3 stalks)
- Lemon (1)

Method for Preparation:
1. Peel the lemon. Remove the core and slice the pears and apples.
2. Toss each of the components into a juicer.

3. Remove the juice and pour it into two chilled glasses to serve.

Meal 1: Spring Onion & Asparagus Frittata: 464

Time Required: 40-45 minutes
Servings: 2
Nutritional Calories: 464

Ingredients Needed:

- Egg (5)
- Almond milk (3 fl. oz./80 ml)
- Coconut oil (2 tbsp.)
- Garlic (1 clove)
- Asparagus tips (100g)
- Spring onions (4)
- Chili flakes (1 pinch)
- Tarragon (1 tsp.)

Method for Preparation:

1. Warm the oven at 430° Fahrenheit/220° Celsius.
2. Chop the onions and mince the garlic.
3. Whisk the eggs, salt, pepper, and milk.
4. Prepare a cast-iron skillet with one tablespoon of oil to heat. Sauté the asparagus, onion, and garlic.
5. Transfer the veggies to a bowl and melt the remainder of the oil in the skillet.
6. Mix in the egg mixture and half of the entire batch of veggies. Pop the pan in the oven to solidify the egg (15 min.).
7. Remove the pan, and add the remainder of the veggies. Bake the meal for another 15 minutes.
8. Sprinkle with the chili flakes and tarragon to serve.

Meal 2: Salmon Burgers: 329

Time Required: 35 minutes
Servings: 5
Nutritional Calories: 329

Ingredients Needed:
The Burgers:
- Olive oil (1 tsp.)
- Fresh kale - ribs removed & chopped (1 cup)
- Shallots (.33 cup)
- Black pepper & salt (as desired)
- Cooked quinoa (.75 cup)
- Skinless salmon fillets (16 oz.)
- Dijon mustard (2 tbsp.)
- Large egg (1)

The Salad:
- Olive oil (2.5 tbsp.)
- Black pepper & salt (as desired)
- Red wine vinegar (2.5 tbsp.)
- Fresh baby arugula (8 cups)
- Halved cherry tomatoes (2 cups)

Method for Preparation:
1. Prepare the burgers in a large wok using the medium temperature setting.
2. Finely chop the shallots, and toss in the oil with the kale, pepper, and salt.
3. Sauté them for about four to five minutes and dump them into a large container.
4. Cool them slightly while you chop four ounces of the salmon into a bowl with the kale mixture.
5. Toss the rest of the salmon into a food processor. Pulse it until it's finely chopped. Toss it into the bowl with the kale.
6. Add the rest of the fixings and shape them into five patties.
7. Warm the wok (medium temp) and cook for about four to five minutes on each side.
8. Prepare the dressing by combining the pepper, salt, shallots, vinegar, and oil.
9. Add in the tomatoes and arugula. Toss and serve with one patty per serving.

Meal 2: Side Dish: Baked Potatoes With Spicy Chickpea Stew: 322
Time Required: 1 hour 10 minutes

Servings: 4-6
Nutritional Calories: 322

Ingredients Needed:

- Baking potatoes - pierced all over (4-6)
- Olive oil (2 tbsp.)
- Red onions (2)
- Cloves garlic (4)
- Ginger (2 cm/0.8-inch)
- Turmeric (2 tbsp.)
- Chili flakes (.5-2 tsp.)
- Cumin seeds (2 tbsp.)
- Water (1 splash or as needed)
- Chopped tomatoes (400g/14 oz. tins - 2 each)
- Cacao/unsweetened cocoa powder (2 tbsp.)
- Kidney/chickpeas ~ with juices (2 x 400g/14 oz. tins)
- Bell peppers - Yellow/your choice of color (2)
- Parsley (2 tbsp. + more to garnish)

Optional - add the calories:

- Salt
- Black pepper
- Side salad

Method for Preparation:

1. Warm the oven at 390° Fahrenheit/200° Celsius.
2. In the meantime, prepare all your ingredients. Pierce the potatoes. Chop the peppers into bite-sized pieces. Mince the ginger, onions, and garlic.
3. Place the potatoes in the heated oven for about one hour.
4. Prepare a saucepan to heat the oil. Add the onion to sauté for five minutes with the lid on until the onions are softened - not browned.
5. Mince and toss in the ginger, cumin, garlic, and chili. Simmer the mixture for about one minute using the low-temperature setting. Mix in the turmeric and a splash of water. Simmer for one more minute.
6. Dump in the tomatoes, cocoa powder/cacao), chickpeas (with liquids), and bell pepper.
7. Wait for it to boil and adjust the temperature setting to low. Simmer until the sauce is thickened (45 min.).
8. Lastly, stir in salt, pepper, and two tablespoons of parsley.
9. Serve the stew over the baked potatoes as desired.

Day 7: 1541 Calories

Green Juice 1: Sirtfood Green Juice: 120
Enjoy that morning juice!

Green Juice 2: Orange & Kale Juice: 315
Time Required: 10 minutes
Servings: 2
Nutritional Calories: 315

Ingredients Needed:

- Oranges (5 large)
- Fresh kale (2)

Method for Preparation:

1. Peel and break the orange into sections. Rinse the kale.
2. Add all of the fixings into a juicer and extract it accordingly.
3. Serve in two glasses when it's ready.

Meal 1: Chilaquiles With Gochujang: 484
Time Required: 50-55 minutes
Servings: 2
Nutritional Calories: 484

Ingredients Needed:

- Ancho chili (1 dried)
- Water (2 cups)
- Squashed tomatoes (1 cup)
- Garlic (2 cloves)
- Salt (1 tsp.)
- Gochujang (.5 tbsp.)
- Tortilla chips (5-6 cups)
- Large eggs (3)
- Olive oil (1 tbsp.)

Method for Preparation:

1. Heat the water and mix in the chili. Simmer it for approximately 15 minutes.
2. Use tongs and remove the chili reserving the water.
3. Combine the chile, one cup of hot water, salt, garlic, tomatoes, and

gochujang.
4. Dumb the sauce into a container to warm for four to five minutes.
5. Mix the chips to cover the sauce.
6. In another skillet, add oil and fry the eggs, sunny-side up.
7. Consider topping - using the chips with eggs, cotija, cilantro, onions, jalapenos, avocado, and onions. Add any extra calories.
8. Serve.

Meal 2: Cauliflower Couscous & Turkey Steak: 462
Time Required: 50-55 minutes
Servings: 2
Nutritional Calories: 462

Ingredients Needed:
- Cauliflower (150g/5.25 oz.)
- Garlic (1 clove)
- Red onion (40g/1.5 oz.)
- Fresh ginger (1 tsp.)
- Bird's eye chili (1)
- Olive oil (2 tbsp.)
- Ground turmeric (2 tsp.)
- Parsley (3/8 oz./10g)
- Dried sage (1 tsp.)
- Sun-dried tomatoes (1 oz./30g)
- Turkey steak (5.25 oz./150g)
- Capers (1 tbsp.)
- Juice (half of 1 lemon)

Method for Preparation:
1. Roughly chop the cauliflower in a food processor until it is similar to breadcrumbs. Finely chop the garlic, onion, dried tomatoes, and chili.
2. Warm one teaspoon of the oil in a skillet. Sauté the ginger, garlic, onion, and chili for two to three minutes. Add the cauliflower and turmeric and sauté for one to two minutes. Take the pan from the burner and add half of the parsley and all of the tomatoes.
3. Prepare the turkey steak with oil and sage.
4. Warm a skillet using the medium temperature setting and cook the steak for about five minutes, flipping as needed for your taste.

5. Drizzle it with juice, capers, and a splash of water. Stir and serve it with the couscous.

Meal 2: Dessert: Berry Smoothie: 160
Time Required: 2-3 minutes
Servings: 2
Nutritional Calories: 160

Ingredients Needed:
- Ripe banana (1)
- Blueberries (100g)
- Blackberries (100g)
- Natural yogurt (2 tbsp.)
- Mild olive oil (30ml)

Method for Preparation:
1. Measure and toss each of the fixings into a mixer/food processor.
2. Mix until smooth and serve them in chilled glasses.

Chapter 4: Phase 2: Day 8-14

This phase is designed for you to steadily drop the pounds - not maintain your current weight. You will have one green juice and three meals from the Sirtfood Diet.

According to Healthline.com, there is no calorie limit in this phase. However, according to the United States Department of Health, adult males typically require 2,000 to 3000 calories daily to maintain weight. Adult females need approximately 1,600 to 2,400 calories per day. However, the amounts will differ depending on activity levels and your age. Others suggest the daily calorie limit is 1500, so eat what is comfortable for you. The calories are calculated for you in this segment also.

Day 8: 1 Green Juice & 3 Meals - 1196 Calories

Daily Juice: Celery Juice: 32
Time Required: 10 minutes
Servings: 2
Nutritional Calories: 32

Ingredients Needed:

- Filtered water (.5 cup)
- Salt (1 pinch)
- Fresh ginger (2 tbsp.)
- Celery stalks with leaves (8)
- Lemon (1 splash/to taste)

Method for Preparation:
1. Peel the ginger and lemon.
2. Toss each of the fixings into a blender and puree until well mixed.
3. Use a mesh strainer to prepare the juice.
4. Serve in two chilled glasses promptly for the best results.

Meal 1: Moroccan Spiced Eggs: 394
Time Required: 50 minutes
Servings: 2
Nutritional Calories: 394

Ingredients Needed:
- Shallot (1)
- Bell pepper - red (1)
- Garlic clove (1)
- Courgette/zucchini (1)
- Olive oil (1 tsp.)
- Mild chili powder (.5 tsp.)
- Ground cinnamon (.25 tsp.)
- Tomato paste/puree (1 tbsp.)
- Ground cumin (.25 tsp.)
- Salt (.5 tsp.)
- Chopped tomatoes (400g/14 oz. can)
- Chickpeas in water (400g/14 oz. can)
- Flat-leaf parsley (10g/3 oz./ small handful)
- Unchilled eggs (4 medium)

Method for Preparation:
1. Peel and finely chop the shallot, zucchini, garlic, parsley, and deseeded bell pepper.
2. Warm a saucepan and add the oil. Toss in the shallot and pepper. Sauté them gently for about five minutes. Add the courgette/zucchini and garlic. Cook for another minute or two. Mix in the tomato puree/paste, spices, and salt.
3. Pour in the chopped tomatoes and chickpeas (soaking liquid too).
4. Raise the temperature setting to medium. With the lid off the pan, simmer the sauce for 30 minutes, reducing in volume by about one-third.
5. Transfer the pan from the burner and fold in the chopped parsley.

6. Set the oven at 35o° Fahrenheit/200° Celsius or with a fan @ 180° Celsius/356° Fahrenheit.
7. When you are ready to cook the eggs, heat the tomato sauce to a gentle simmer and transfer them into a small oven-proof dish.
8. Crack the eggs on the side of the dish and lower them gently into the stew.
9. Use a layer of aluminum foil to cover the pan. Set a timer and bake them for 10 to 15 minutes.
10. Serve the mixture using individual bowls with the eggs floating on the top.

Meal 2: Tuna - Egg & Caper Salad: 309

Time Required: 20-25 minutes
Servings: 2
Nutritional Calories: 309

Ingredients Needed:

- Red/yellow chicory (3.5 oz.)
- Tuna flakes in brine (5 oz. can)
- Rocket arugula (1 oz.)
- Cucumber (3.5 oz.)
- Black olives (6 pitted)
- Tomatoes (2)
- Hard-boiled eggs (2)
- Red onion (1)
- Fresh parsley (2 tbsp.)
- Celery (1 stalk)
- Capers (1 tbsp.)
- Garlic vinaigrette - see the recipe below (2 tbsp.)

Method for Preparation:

1. Drain the tuna. Cook, peel, and quarter the eggs. Chop the tomatoes, onions, and parsley.
2. Combine the olives, cucumber, tuna, onion, celery, chicory, parsley, and arugula in a salad bowl.
3. Add the vinaigrette and toss.
4. Serve and garnish with the capers and eggs.

Meal 3: Fried Chicken & Broccolini: 461
Time Required: 45 minutes
Servings: 2
Nutritional Calories: 461

Ingredients Needed:

- Coconut oil (2 tbsp.)
- Chicken breast (14 oz./400g)
- Bacon cubes (5.25 oz. /250g)
- Broccolini (8 oz. /250g)

Method for Preparation:

1. Slice the chicken into cubes.
2. Prepare a skillet with oil and heat using the medium temperature setting.
3. Add the chicken and bacon with a sprinkle of salt, pepper, and chili flakes.
4. Toss in the broccolini and continue to cook until done to your liking.
5. Stack on two plates and enjoy or save one for the next day.

Day 9: 1 Green Juice & 3 Meals - 1466 Calories

Daily Juice: Celery Juice: 32
Time Required: 10 minutes
Servings: 2
Nutritional Calories: 32

Ingredients Needed:

- Celery stalks with leaves (8)
- Fresh ginger (2 tbsp.)
- Lemon (1)
- Filtered water (.5 cup)
- Salt (1 pinch)

Method for Preparation:

1. Peel the lemon and ginger.
2. Toss each of the fixings into a blender and thoroughly puree until incorporated.
3. Strain the juice using a mesh strainer.

4. Serve in two glasses right away.

Meal 1: Chocolate Muffins: 410

Time Required: 35 minutes
Servings: 6
Nutritional Calories: 410

Ingredients Needed:

- Buckwheat flour (.5 cup)
- Almond flour (.5 cup)
- Cacao powder (4 tbsp.)
- Arrowroot powder (4 tbsp.)
- Baking powder (1 tsp.)
- Bicarbonate soda (.5 tsp.)
- Boiling water (.5 cup)
- Maple syrup (.33 cup)
- Melted coconut oil (.33 cup)
- Apple cider vinegar (1 tbsp.)
- Unsweetened dark chocolate chips (.5 cup)

Method for Preparation:

1. Warm the oven at 350° Fahrenheit/177° Celsius.
2. Prepare six muffin tin cups with paper liners.
3. Whisk both of the flours, baking powder, arrowroot powder, and bicarbonate soda.
4. In another container, whisk the syrup, boiled water, and oil. Combine with the flour until just mixed and fold in the chips of chocolate.
5. Add the prepared batter to the cups and set a timer to bake them for 20 minutes.
6. Let them cool in the tin on a rack for about ten minutes.
7. Invert the semi-cooled muffins to a rack to cool before serving.

Meal 1: Kale & Blackcurrant Smoothie: 86

Time Required: 3-5 minutes
Servings: 2
Nutritional Calories: 86

Ingredients Needed:

- Honey (2 tsp.)
- Freshly brewed green tea (1 cup)
- Ripe banana (1)
- Blackcurrants (40 g)
- Baby kale (10 leaves)
- Ice (6 cubes)

Method for Preparation:

1. Remove the stalks from the kale. Wash and remove the stalks from the blackcurrants.
2. Mix the green tea and honey until dissolved.
3. Combine each of the fixings into a blender until they're creamy smooth. Serve immediately.

Meal 2: Chargrilled Beef with Onion Rings, Kale, & Potatoes 240

Time Required: 1 hour 15 minutes
Servings: 2
Nutritional Calories: 240

Ingredients Needed:

- Potatoes (100g/3.5 oz.)
- Olive oil (1 tbsp.)
- Parsley (3/5g/316 oz.)
- Red onion (50g/1 ⅝ oz.)
- Kale (50g/1 ⅝ oz.)
- Garlic clove (1)
- Thick beef fillet steak (4 @ 5.75 oz. x 3.5cm) or sirloin steak (.25-inch x 2cm-thick) - Your choice
- Red wine (40ml/1.35 fl. oz.)
- Tomato purée (1 tsp.)
- Beef stock (150ml/4 fl. oz.)
- Cornflour (1 tsp.) dissolved in water (1 tbsp.)

Method for Preparation:

1. Heat the oven at 220°Celsius/428° Fahrenheit.
2. Finely chop the garlic and parsley. Slice the onion into rings and coarsely slice the kale.
3. Peel, dice (2 cm size), and toss the potatoes in a saucepan of boiling

water. Once they are boiling, set a timer for five minutes and drain. Put them in a roasting pan with one teaspoon of the oil to roast (35-45 min.).

4. Flip the potatoes every ten minutes. Transfer them from the oven, sprinkle with parsley, and stir.
5. Sauté the onion in one teaspoon of oil using the medium temperature setting for five to seven minutes, until caramelized. Keep warm.
6. Steam the kale for two to three minutes and drain.
7. Sauté the garlic gently in ½ teaspoon of oil for one minute, until softened, but not colored. Fold in the kale and sauté them for another one to two minutes. Keep warm.
8. Warm an oven-proof skillet using the high-temperature setting until it's smoking hot. Baste the beef using ½ a teaspoon of the oil.
9. Place the meat into the hot skillet and fry using the med-high temperature setting until it's as you like it.
10. Transfer the meat from the pan to a platter for now.
11. Dump the wine into the hot skillet to dislodge the browned bits. Simmer to reduce the wine until it's concentrated and syrupy.
12. Pour in the tomato purée and stock to the steak pan. Wait for it to boil and mix in the cornflour paste, adding it a little at a time to thicken.
13. Stir in the juices from the steak platter.
14. Serve the meat with the onion rings, kale, roasted potatoes, and wine sauce.

Meal 3: Spinach & Eggplant Casserole 446

Time Required: 1 hour
Servings: 2
Nutritional Calories: 446

Ingredients Needed:

- Eggplant (1)
- Onion (2)
- Olive oil (3 tbsp.)
- Fresh spinach (16 oz./450g)
- Tomatoes (4)
- Eggs (2)
- Almond milk (60 ml/2 fl. oz.)
- Lemon juice (2 tsp.)
- Almond flour (4 tbsp.)

Method for Preparation:

1. Warm the oven to reach 390° Fahrenheit/200° Celsius. Lightly grease a baking tray.
2. Slice the onions, eggplant, and tomatoes. Sprinkle them with salt.
3. Lightly brush the onions and eggplant with oil and add them to a grill pan.
4. Shrink the spinach in a saucepan using the medium temperature setting. Drain it in a sieve.
5. Arrange the veggies in layers on the baking sheet; eggplant, spinach, onion, and tomato. Repeat the layer.
6. Whisk the eggs, milk, pepper, salt, and lemon juice. Pour it over the vegetables.
7. Sprinkle the flour over the dish. Bake the delicious meal for 30-40 minutes.

Meal 3: Snack or Dessert: Buckwheat Granola 252

Time Required: 45 minutes
Servings: 10
Nutritional Calories: 252

Ingredients Needed:

- Olive oil (2 tbsp.)
- Buckwheat groats (2 cups)
- Ground ginger (1 tsp.)
- Cinnamon (1 tsp.)
- Chopped almonds (.75 cup)
- Pumpkin seeds (.75 cup)
- Coconut flakes (1 cup - unsweetened)
- Banana (1 ripe)
- Maple syrup (2 tbsp.)

Method for Preparation:

1. Peel the banana and chop the almonds.
2. Warm the oven to reach 350° Fahrenheit/ 177° Celsius.
3. Toss the buckwheat in a container with the spices, almonds, seeds, and coconut flakes.
4. In another container, mix the banana.
5. Mix the buckwheat mix, oil, and maple syrup. Combine everything and place it on the baking tray (single-layered).
6. Bake the granola for 25-30 minutes. Stir about halfway through the

cooking cycle.

7. Cool before serving.

Day 10: 1 Green Juice & 3 Meals - 1543 Calories

Daily Juice: Broccoli - Apple & Orange Juice: 254
Time Required: 10 minutes
Servings: 2
Nutritional Calories: 254

Ingredients Needed:

- Broccoli (2 stalks)
- Sliced green apples (2 large)
- Oranges (3 large)
- Fresh parsley (4 tbsp.)

Method for Preparation:

1. Core the apples and chop the broccoli. Peel and section the oranges.
2. Toss all of the components into a juicer and extract the juice.
3. Pour and serve in two glasses to serve right away for the best flavor.

Meal 1: Chinese Pork With Choi: 377
Time Required: 15-20 minutes
Servings: 4
Nutritional Calories: 377

Ingredients Needed:

- Firm tofu (400g)
- Water (1 tbsp.)
- Cornflour (1 tbsp.)
- Rice wine (1 tbsp.)
- Chicken stock (125 ml)
- Tomato purée (1 tbsp.)
- Brown sugar (1 tsp.)
- Soy sauce (1 tbsp.)
- Garlic (1 clove)
- Fresh ginger (1 thumb/5cm)

- Rapeseed oil (1 tbsp.)
- Shiitake mushrooms (100g)
- Shallot (1)
- Pak Choi/Choi sum (200g)
- Minced pork - 10% fat (400g)
- Bean sprouts (100g)
- Parsley (20g/1 large handful)

Method for Preparation:

1. Peel and slice the shallot and Choi. Chop the parsley and tofu (large chunks).
2. Place the tofu on a layer of parchment baking paper. Cover with another sheet of paper.
3. Whisk the cornflour and water to remove all of the lumps. Pour in the chicken stock, tomato purée, rice wine, soy sauce, and brown sugar. Mince and fold in the ginger and garlic.
4. Prepare a wok or large skillet to warm the oil using the high-temperature setting. Slice and mix in the mushrooms. Stir-fry them for two to three minutes.
5. Transfer the mushrooms from the pan into a container.
6. Place the tofu in the pan and stir-fry until it's golden. Transfer it to a container for now.
7. Add the pak choi and shallots to the wok, stir-fry for two minutes, and add it to the mince. Simmer until done and add the sauce. Reduce the temperature setting and cook for a minute or two.
8. Fold in the tofu, sprouts, and mushrooms to warm thoroughly.
9. Transfer the pan to the countertop, garnish it using the parsley and serve promptly.

Meal 2: Horseradish-Flaked Salmon Fillet & Kale: 206

Time Required: 35-40 minutes
Servings: 2
Nutritional Calories: 206

Ingredients Needed:

- Olive oil (1 tbsp.)
- Boneless-skinless salmon fillet (7 oz./200g)
- Green beans (1 5/8 oz./50g)
- Kale (2.25 oz./75g)
- Garlic (half of 1 clove)

- Red onion (1 ⅝ oz./50g)
- Flat-leaf parsley (1 tbsp.)
- Fresh chives (1 tbsp.)
- Horseradish sauce (1 tbsp.)
- Low-fat creme fraiche (1 tbsp.)
- Juice (1.4 of 1 lemon)
- Black pepper & salt
- Also Needed: Steamer basket

Method for Preparation:

1. Mince the garlic. Chop the parsley, chives, and onion.
2. Warm the grill.
3. Dust the fillet with pepper and salt. Grill it for 10 to 15 minutes. Flake it into a container and set it aside for now.
4. Steam the green beans and kale for ten minutes.
5. Warm the oil in a skillet using the high-temperature setting.
6. Toss in the onion and garlic. Fry them for two to three minutes. Toss in the beans and kale. Sauté for another one to two minutes.
7. Mix the salmon, juice, horseradish, parsley, chives, and creme fraiche.
8. Serve the beans and kale with the delicious salmon.

Meal 3: Kale & Feta Salad With Cranberry Dressing: 706

Time Required: 30-35 minutes
Servings: 2
Nutritional Calories: 706

Ingredients Needed:

- Kale (9 oz.)
- Walnuts (2 oz.)
- Feta cheese (3 oz.)
- Apple (1)
- Medjool dates (4)

The Dressing:

- Water (3 tbsp.)
- Red onion (half of 1)
- Cranberries (3 oz.)
- Red wine vinegar (1 tbsp.)
- Olive oil (3 tbsp.)
- Honey (2 tsp.)

- Sea salt

Method for Preparation:

1. Finely chop the kale, dates, onion, parsley, and walnuts.
2. Core, peel, and slice the apple. Crumble the feta.
3. Toss the dressing fixings in a food processor. Pulse them until they're creamy, adding water as needed.
4. Add each of the fixings to a salad bowl. Pour the dressing and gently toss before serving.

Day 11: 1 Green Juice & 3 Meals - 1510 Calories

Daily Juice: Kale - Carrot & Grapefruit Juice: 232
Time Required: 10 minutes
Servings: 2
Nutritional Calories: 232

Ingredients Needed:

- Grapefruit (2 medium)
- Carrots (2)
- Fresh kale (3 cups)
- Granny Smith apple (2 large)
- Fresh juice (1 tsp./1 lemon)

Method for Preparation:

1. Remove the peelings from the grapefruit and carrots. Slice and core the apple. Section the grapefruit, and squeeze the juice. Roughly chop the carrots.
2. Toss the prepared fixings into the juicer.
3. Extract the juice and pour it into two chilled glasses and serve.

Meal 1: Apple Pancakes With Blackcurrant Compote: 337
Time Required: 40-45 minutes
Servings: 6
Nutritional Calories: 337

Ingredients Needed:

- Coconut sugar (2 tbsp.)
- Ground cinnamon (.5 tsp.)
- Buckwheat flour (.5 cup)
- Baking powder (1 tsp.)
- Unsweetened almond milk (.33 cup)
- Egg (1)
- Granny Smith apples (2)

Method for Preparation:

1. Whisk the cinnamon with the sugar and flour into a mixing container.
2. Core, peel, and grate the apples.
3. Whisk the egg and milk in another container.
4. Combine the dry and wet fixings, and mix in the apples.
5. Warm a wok using the med-high temperature setting. Spoon in the mixture.
6. Cook each side for one to two minutes. Continue until you have six portions.
7. Serve with a drizzle of warm honey.

Meal 2: Sweet & Sour Pan With Cashew Nuts: 573

Time Required: ½ hour
Servings: 2
Nutritional Calories: 573

Ingredients Needed:

- Arrowroot powder (2 tsp.)
- Coconut oil (2 tbsp.)
- Red onion (2 pieces)
- Pak/bok choy (150g/5.25 oz.)
- Yellow pepper (2 pieces)
- White cabbage (250g/9 oz.)
- Mung bean sprouts (1 ⅝ oz./50g)
- Pineapple slices (4)
- Cashew nuts (1 ⅝ oz./50g)

The Sauce:

- Apple cider vinegar (2 fl. oz./60 ml)
- Coconut blossom sugar (4 tbsp.)

- Tomato paste (2 tbsp.)
- Water (75 ml/2.5 fl.oz.)
- Coconut amino (1 tsp.)

Method for Preparation:

1. Roughly chop the veggies and mix the arrowroot with five tablespoons of water to make a paste.
2. Toss the rest of the fixings into a saucepan and mix in the paste.
3. Melt the oil in a skillet and sauté the onion. Toss in the pak choy, cabbage, bell pepper, and sprouts.
4. Stir-fry the veggies until they're softened.
5. Fold in the pineapple and cashews.
6. Serve with a portion of sauce.

Meal 3: Prawns & Asparagus: 253 & Braised Leek & Pine Nuts: 115

Time Required: 28-30 minutes
Servings: 4
Nutritional Calories: 253

Ingredients Needed:

- Prawns (1 lb.)
- Olive oil (3 tbsp.)
- Black pepper & salt (to your liking)
- Garlic (1 tsp.)
- Fresh ginger (1 tsp.)
- Asparagus (1 lb.)
- Soy sauce - low-sodium (1 tbsp.)
- Lemon juice (2 tbsp.)

Method for Preparation:

1. Peel and devein the shrimp. Mince the ginger and garlic, and trim the asparagus.
2. Prepare a wok with two tablespoons of oil using the med-high heat setting.
3. Toss in the prawns, salt, and pepper to sauté for about three to four minutes.
4. Scoop them into a bowl and set to the side for now.
5. Warm the rest of the oil (1 tbsp.) using the same heat setting. Toss in the ginger, asparagus, black pepper, and salt. Sauté them for six to eight minutes, stirring often.
6. Fold in the prawns with the soy sauce and sauté them for about one

minute.

7. Spritz them with the lemon juice, remove from the burner and serve.

Day 12: 1 Green Juice & 3 Meals - 1486 Calories

Daily Juice: Celery Juice: 32
Time Required: 10 minutes
Servings: 2
Nutritional Calories: 32

Ingredients Needed:

- Celery stalks with leaves (8)
- Fresh ginger (2 tbsp.)
- Lemon (1)
- Filtered water (.5 cup)
- Salt (1 pinch)

Method for Preparation:

1. Peel the lemon and ginger.
2. Toss each of the fixings into a blender. Pulse until they are thoroughly pureed and incorporated. Strain the juice using a mesh strainer.
3. Serve in two glasses while it's fresh.

Meal 1: Buckwheat Pancakes: 240
Time Required: ½ hour
Servings: 6 cakes
Nutritional Calories: 240
Ingredients Needed:

- Buckwheat flour (60g/.5 cup)
- Baking powder - double-acting (.5 tsp.)
- Natural sweetener - ex. stevia/etc. (2-4 packets /as desired)
- Salt (1/8 tsp.)
- Unsweetened vanilla almond milk/your choice (.5 cup)

Method for Preparation:

1. Warm a pancake griddle using the medium temperature setting. Lightly spritz the grids using cooking oil spray.

2. Whisk the flour with the sweetener of choice, baking powder, and salt. Mix in the milk.
3. Pour the batter into the heated griddle. Cook them for two to four minutes. Flip the pancakes when they have bubbled on the first side. Cook them for another two to four minutes. Do this until all batter is gone.

Meal 2: Beef With Carrots & Kale: 311

Time Required: 27 minutes to ½ hour
Servings: 4
Nutritional Calories: 311

Ingredients Needed:

- Garlic cloves (4)
- Carrots (1.5 cups)
- Fresh kale (1.5 cups)
- Coconut oil (2 tbsp.)
- Sirloin beef steak (1 lb.)
- Ground black pepper (to your liking)
- Tamari (3 tbsp.)

Method for Preparation:

1. Mince the garlic. Peel and slice the carrots into matchsticks, and remove the tough ribs from the kale.
2. Melt the oil in a wok using the medium-temperature setting. Toss in and sauté the garlic (1 min.), add in the beef and pepper. Adjust the temperature setting to med-high. Cook the meat for three to four minutes until browned.
3. Toss in the tamari, kale, and carrots. Sauté them for about four to five minutes.
4. Remove and serve them hot.

Meal 2: Side Dish: Twice Baked Potatoes: 647

Time Required: 2 hours 10 minutes
Servings: 2
Nutritional Calories: 647

Ingredients Needed:

- Reddish-brown potatoes (2 medium)

- Black pepper and salt (as desired)
- Unsalted margarine spread (2 tbsp.)
- Cooked bacon (4 rashers)
- Heavy cream (3 tbsp.)
- Large eggs (4)
- Shredded cheddar (.5 cup)
- Chives (as desired)

Method for Preparation:

1. Wash the potatoes and poke holes in them with a fork.
2. Warm a grill/oven at 400° Fahrenheit/204° Celsius.
3. Place the potatoes in the center of the rack and cook for 30-45 minutes.
4. Transfer them to the countertop to cool for about 15 minutes.
5. Slice them lengthwise and remove the potato from the skin into a mixing container.
6. Add the spread, salt, pepper, and cream to the white potatoes, mixing until creamy. Scoop a portion of the mixture back into the potatoes and garnish with cheese. Add a slice of bacon to each half and top with an egg.
7. Pop them in the oven to broil at 375° Fahrenheit/191° Celsius until the whites are done, and the yolk is runny. Top them using the rest of the cheese.
8. Serve with a sprinkle of chives as desired.

Meal 3: Buckwheat Noodles With Chicken - Kale & Miso Dressing: 256

Time Required: ½ hour
Servings: 2
Nutritional Calories: 256

Ingredients Needed:
The Noodles:

- Kale leaves (2-3 handfuls)
- Buckwheat noodles (100% buckwheat - no wheat (150g/ 5 oz.)
- Shiitake mushrooms (3-4)
- Coconut oil or ghee (1 tsp.)
- Brown onion (1)
- Free-range chicken breast (1 medium)
- Red chili (1 long)
- Garlic cloves (2 large)

- Tamari sauce/Soy sauce - Gluten-free preferred (2-3 tbsp.)

For the Dressing:

- Olive oil (1 tbsp.)
- Tamari sauce (1 tbsp.)
- Fresh organic miso (1.5 tbsp.)
- Lime or lemon juice (1 tbsp.)
- Sesame oil (1 tsp.)

Method for Preparation:

1. Slice or dice the chicken. Slice the mushrooms and chili. Finely dice the onion and garlic.
2. Prepare a medium saucepan of water and wait for it to boil. Remove the stems, and add the kale to the pot to cook for one minute, until it's slightly wilted. Remove and set it aside, but reserve the water and wait for it to boil again.
3. Fold in the noodles and cook per the packet directions (5 min.). Rinse them in a colander using cold water and set them aside to drain.
4. Sprinkle the mushrooms with salt and pan-fry it in ghee/coconut oil (1 tsp.) for two to three minutes, until lightly browned on each side. Set them aside.
5. In the same skillet, warm more oil/ghee using the med-high temperature setting. Sauté the onion and chili for two to three minutes, and then add in the pieces of chicken. Simmer the mixture for about five minutes using a medium-temperature setting. Mix in the garlic, tamari sauce, and a sprinkle of water. Simmer for about two to three minutes, often stirring until the chicken is thoroughly done.
6. Lastly, add the soba noodles and kale. Toss them with the chicken to heat.
7. Whisk the dressing. Sprinkle it over the noodles during the last minute of the cooking cycle and serve.

Day 13: 1 Green Juice & 3 Meals - 1497 Calories

Daily Juice: Sirtfood Green Juice: 120

Time Required: 10-15minutes

Servings: 2

Nutritional Calories: 120

Ingredients Needed:

- Celery (150g - including leaves/2-3 large stalks)

- Kale (75g/2 large handfuls)
- Arugula (30g/1 large handful)
- Flat-leaf parsley (5g/1 small handful)
- Optional: Lovage leaves (5g/1 small handful)*
- Green apple (half of 1 medium)
- Lemon juice (half of 1 lemon)
- Matcha green tea (.5 level tsp.)

Method for Preparation:

1. Mix the greens (parsley, rocket, lovage, and kale) and juice them to provide about 50ml/.21 cup of juice.
2. Juice the apple and celery. Peel the lemon by hand - not a knife. You should have about one cup of juice or maybe more.
3. Add the tea when it's time to serve. Pour a small portion into a serving glass and mix in the matcha. After the matcha has dissolved, combine it with the rest of the juice.
4. Pour it into two glasses and serve immediately.

Meal 1: Mexican Egg-Filled Bell Peppers: 497

Time Required: 55 minutes
Servings: 2
Nutritional Calories: 497

Ingredients Needed:

- Coconut oil (1 tbsp.)
- Egg (4)
- Tomato (1)
- Chili flakes (1 pinch)
- Ground cumin (.25 tsp.)
- Paprika (.25 tsp.)
- Green peppers (1)
- Avocado (half of 1)
- Fresh coriander (2 tbsp.)

Method for Preparation:

1. Slice the bell pepper into half. Slice the avocado and tomatoes into cubes. Finely chop the coriander.
2. Melt the oil in a skillet using the medium temperature setting.
3. Whisk the eggs with salt, pepper, paprika, caraway, and chili.

4. Add the avocado and put the egg mixture into each of the pepper halves and garnish with the coriander.

Meal 2: Sesame Chicken Salad: 304

Time Required: 12-15 minutes
Servings: 2
Nutritional Calories: 304

Ingredients Needed:

- Cucumber (1)
- Baby kale (100g)
- Sesame seeds (1 tbsp.)
- Pak choi (60g pkg.)
- Parsley (1 large handful /20g)
- Red onion (half of 1)
- Cooked chicken (150g)

The Dressing:

- Sesame oil (1 tsp.)
- Soy sauce (2 tsp.)
- Clear honey (1 tsp.)
- Olive oil (1 tbsp.)
- Juice of 1 lime

Method for Preparation:

1. Prepare the cucumber by peeling and slicing it in half lengthways. Roughly chop the kale. Deseed the cucumber with a teaspoon and slice it. Finely shred the onion, Choi, and chicken. Chop the parsley.
2. Toast the sesame seeds in a dry skillet until lightly browned (2 min.). Once fragrant, scoop them onto a platter until cooled.
3. Prepare the dressing by whisking the olive and sesame oil with the honey, lime juice, and soy sauce.
4. Arrange the pak choi, kale, red onion, cucumber, and parsley in a serving salad bowl. Toss gently. Dump the dressing over the salad and toss again.
5. Portion the salad into two plates.
6. Top them using the shredded chicken and sesame seeds at serving time.

Meal 2: Side Dish: Greek Salad Skewers: 306
Time Required: 10 minutes
Servings: 2
Nutritional Calories: 306

Ingredients Needed:
- Wooden skewers (2)
- Yellow pepper (1 cut into 8 squares)
- Cherry tomatoes (8)
- Red onion (half of 1 - separated into 8 pieces)
- Large black olives (8)
- Cucumber (100g/about 10 cm - cut into 4 slices & halved)
- Feta (100g - cut into 8 cubes)

For the Dressing:
- Clove garlic (half of 1)
- Basil & oregano (several leaves of each) or Dried mixed herbs (.5 tsp.)
- Olive oil (1 tbsp. of extra-virgin)
- Balsamic vinegar (1 tsp.)
- Juice of ½ lemon
- Black pepper and salt (as desired)
- Also Needed: Skewers

Method for Preparation:
1. Soak the wooden skewers for ½ hour before using.
2. Peel and mince the garlic. Finely chop the oregano and basil.
3. Thread each of the skewers with the salad fixings in the following order: Olives, tomatoes, yellow peppers, red onions, cucumbers, feta, tomatoes, olives, yellow peppers, red onions, cucumbers, and feta.
4. Toss all the dressing fixings and mix them thoroughly. Dump it over the skewers and cook on the grill as desired.

Meal 3: Shrimp & Kale: 270
Time Required: 25 minutes
Servings: 4
Nutritional Calories: 270

Ingredients Needed:
- Olive oil (3 tbsp.)

- Medium shrimp (1 lb.)
- Garlic (4 cloves)
- Medium onion (1)
- Red chili (1 fresh)
- Kale (1 lb.)
- Low-sodium chicken broth

Method for Preparation:

1. Peel and devein the shrimp. Chop the onion, slice the chili, and mince the garlic. Remove the ribs from the kale and chop it to bits.
2. Prepare a wok with one tablespoon of oil and heat it using the med-high temperature setting.
3. Toss in the shrimp to stir fry for about two minutes per side.
4. Remove the shrimp into a bowl.
5. Warm the rest of the oil (2 tbsp.) using the medium temperature setting. Toss in the chili and garlic to sauté for about 60 seconds, stirring intermittently.
6. Stir in the shrimp to reheat for about one minute and serve them hot.

Day 14: 1 Green Juice & 3 Meals - 1441 Calories

Daily Juice: Green Fruit Juice - No Kale: 304
Time Required: 10 minutes
Servings: 2
Nutritional Calories: 304

Ingredients Needed:

- Kiwi (3 large)
- Fresh lime juice (2 tsp.)
- Green apples (3 large)
- Seedless green grapes (2 cups)

Method for Preparation:

1. Peel and chop the kiwi. Slice and core the apples.
2. Toss each of the ingredients into a juicer.
3. Remove the juice and pour it into two glasses to serve.

Meal 1: Gluten-Free Buckwheat Pancakes With Roasted Strawberries: 455
Time Required: 25 minutes
Servings: 2-8 cakes
Nutritional Calories: 455

Ingredients Needed:

- Buckwheat flour (1 cup) or (½ cup each - flour of choice + buckwheat)
- Salt (.25 tsp.)
- Baking powder & soda (1 tsp. of each)
- Sugar (1 tbsp.)
- Buttermilk (1.25 cups - shaken)
- Egg (1 large)
- Pure vanilla extract (.5 tsp.)
- For the skillet: Butter (as needed)

The Berries:

- Sugar (1 tsp.)
- Strawberries (1 pint)
- Maple syrup or honey (1 tbsp.)

Method for Preparation:

1. Hull and slice the strawberries into halves or quarters.
2. Roast the strawberries. Set the oven at 350° Fahrenheit/177 °Celsius.
3. Prepare a rimmed baking tray using a layer of parchment baking paper.
4. Toss the berries with the honey/syrup and sugar.
5. Toss the berries on the baking tray - not touching. Set a timer and roast them for about half an hour. Stir about halfway through the cycle as the berry juices thicken.
6. Whisk the baking soda, salt, flour (s), sugar, and baking powder.
7. Use a liquid measuring cup and add the buttermilk. Whisk in the vanilla and egg.
8. Combine the wet fixings with the dry ones and stir (a few lumps are okay.)
9. Warm a frying pan with 1.5 teaspoons of butter using the med-low temperature setting.
10. Swirl the batter with a spoon in case the buckwheat is starting to separate from the liquid.
11. Scoop the batter onto the warm skillet (¼ cup each). Cook the cakes for two to three minutes until small bubbles form on the surface of the pancakes. Cook until golden brown (1-2 min.).
12. Transfer them to a baking sheet and pop them in a warm oven at 200° Fahrenheit/93° Celsius oven to keep them warm as you finish each

batch.

13. Serve them when ready.

Meal 2: Chicken & Kale Curry: 313

Time Required: 1 hour 50 minutes
Servings: 4
Nutritional Calories: 313

Ingredients Needed:

- Red onions (2)
- Garlic cloves (3)
- Ginger (1 tbsp.)
- Birdseye/Thai chili (2)
- Skinless and boneless chicken thighs (400g)
- Olive oil (1 tbsp.)
- Cardamom pods (2)
- Curry powder (1 tbsp.)
- Ground turmeric (2 tbsp.)
- Coconut milk - light (200 ml tinned)
- Chicken stockpot (1)
- Boiling water (500 ml)
- Chopped tomatoes (175g - tinned)

Method for Preparation:

1. Dice the onions, garlic, ginger, and chili.
2. Place the chicken in a glass/plastic bowl and add one teaspoon of the oil and one tablespoon of the turmeric. Mix well and marinate for ½ hour.
3. Fry the chicken using the medium temperature setting (4-5 min.). Transfer the chicken to a platter and set it on the countertop for now.
4. Warm the rest of the oil using the medium temperature setting. Toss in the onion, chili, garlic, and ginger to sauté until softened (10 min.).
5. Measure and stir in the curry powder and another tablespoon of the turmeric. Simmer for an additional one to two minutes.
6. Pour in the stock, tomatoes, coconut milk, and cardamom pods. Simmer for 30 minutes.
7. When the sauce has reduced a bit, fold in the chicken, followed by the kale. Cook until the chicken has warmed thoroughly, and the kale is tender.
8. Serve with rice or buckwheat. If using buckwheat, simmer it for slightly

less time than recommended on the packet.

9. Garnish with chopped coriander before serving.

Meal 2: Side Dish: Arugula - Strawberry & Orange Salad: 107

Time Required: 15 minutes
Servings: 4
Nutritional Calories: 107

Ingredients Needed:

- Fresh baby arugula (6 cups)
- Oranges (peeled & segmented)
- Fresh strawberries (sliced)

The Dressing:

- Fresh juice from 1 lemon (2 tbsp.)
- Dijon mustard (1 tsp.)
- Raw honey (1 tbsp.)
- Salt & Freshly cracked pepper (as desired)
- Olive oil (2 tsp.)

Method for Preparation:

1. Make the salad and dressing by combining the fixings.
2. Toss it all thoroughly and serve promptly for the best flavor results.

Meal 3: Kale Salad & Beef: 262

Time Required: 24-28 minutes
Servings: 2
Nutritional Calories: 262

Ingredients Needed:

The Steak:

- Strip steaks (2 @ 4 oz. each)
- Olive oil (2 tsp.)
- Freshly cracked pepper and salt (to taste)

The Salad:

- Cucumber (.25 cup)
- Radish (.25 cup)
- Carrot (.25 cup)
- Cherry tomatoes (.25 cup)
- Fresh kale (3 cups)

The Dressing:

- Fresh juice (1 tbsp./1 lemon)

- Olive oil (1 tbsp.)
- Fresh black pepper & salt (as desired)

Method for Preparation:

1. Slice the tomatoes into halves. Peel and shred the carrot. Peel and slice the cucumber and radish. Remove the ribs from the kale and coarsely chop it.
2. Prepare a heavy-bottomed wok to warm the oil using the high-temperature setting. Add the steaks and sprinkle with pepper and salt. Cook about three to four minutes per side.
3. Arrange the steaks on a cutting block and wait about five minutes before slicing.
4. Toss all of the salad fixings into a bowl.
5. Prepare the dressing and slice the steaks against the grain.
6. Portion the fixings and serve with a drizzle of dressing.

Chapter 5: Phase 2: Day 15-21

As you enter into this phase of the Sirtfood diet plan you will continue to have one green juice and three meals to be maintained at around 1500 calories. Keep up the good work!

Day 15: 1 Green Juice & 3 Meals - 1472 Calories

Daily Juice: Grape & Melon Juice: 125
Time Required: 2-3 minutes
Servings: 1
Nutritional Calories: 125

Ingredients Needed:

- Celery stalk (1)
- Green apple (1)
- Kiwis (2)
- Lime (half of 1)
- A pinch of pink Himalayan salt (1 pinch)
- Turmeric (.5 tsp.)
- Organic honey (.5 tbsp.)

Method for Preparation:

1. Chop the celery, kiwis, and apple.
2. Toss each of the fixings into a blender.

3. Thoroughly mix and pour into a cold glass.

Meal 1: Chocolate Waffles: 295
Time Required: 40-45 minutes
Servings: 8
Nutritional Calories: 295

Ingredients Needed:

- Unsweetened almond milk (2 cups)
- Fresh juice (1 lemon/1 tbsp.)
- Cacao powder (.5 cup)
- Buckwheat flour (1 cup)
- Baking powder (1 tsp.)
- Flaxseed meal (.25 cup)
- Kosher salt (.25 tsp.)
- Baking soda (1 tsp.)
- Large eggs (2)
- Melted coconut oil (.5 cup)
- Dark brown sugar (.25 cup)
- Vanilla extract (2 tsp.)
- Unsweetened dark chocolate (2 oz.)

Method for Preparation:

1. Roughly chop the chocolate. Whisk the juice and almond milk and let it rest (undisturbed) for ten minutes.
2. Whisk/sift the salt, baking powder, flaxseed meal, baking soda, cacao, and flour.
3. Mix the milk fixings, eggs, oil, vanilla, and brown sugar.
4. Fold in the flour mixture, mixing it until it's smooth. Fold in the bits of chocolate.
5. Warm and spritz the waffle iron using cooking oil spray.
6. Pour the batter into the grill and cook for about three minutes. Continue until you have equally prepared eight servings.

Meal 2: Salmon & Spinach Quiche: 903
Time Required: 55 minutes
Servings: 2
Nutritional Calories: 903

Ingredients Needed:

- Frozen leaf spinach (21 oz./600g)
- Garlic (1 clove)
- Onion (1)
- Frozen salmon fillets (5.25 oz./150g)
- Smoked salmon (7 oz./200g)
- Dill (1 small bunch)
- Lemon (1)
- Butter (1 ⅝ oz./50g)
- Sour cream (7 oz./200g)
- Eggs (3)
- Puff pastry (1 pkg.)
- Nutmeg - salt & pepper (as desired)
- Also Needed: Springform pan

Method for Preparation:

1. Thaw and squeeze out the spinach. Rinse, pat dry, and chop the dill.
2. Peel and dice the garlic and onion.
3. Slice the salmon fillet into cubes and the smoked salmon into strips.
4. Rinse the lemon, dry, and grate the zest. Squeeze the juice.
5. Warm the butter in a skillet. Toss in the garlic and onion to sauté for two to three minutes.
6. Mix the juice, zest, eggs, and sour cream with the nutmeg, salt, and pepper.
7. Warm the oven at 390° Fahrenheit/200° Celsius.
8. Grease the pan, roll out the pastry and arrange it to the edges. Dot it using a fork, so it doesn't rise too high.
9. Pour in the egg mixture and smooth it out. Add the salmon cubes and strips on top.
10. Place the quiche on the middle rack of the oven. Set the timer to bake for about 40 minutes until it's golden.

Meal 3: Aromatic Chicken Breast - Kale - Red Onion & Salsa: 149

Time Required: 30-35 minutes
Servings: 1
Nutritional Calories: 149

Ingredients Needed:

- Skinless - boneless chicken breast (120g/4.25 oz.)
- Ground turmeric (2 tsp.)

- Olive oil (1 tbsp.)
- Juice (1/4 of one lemon)
- Kale (50g)
- Red onion (20g)
- Fresh ginger (1 tsp.)
- Buckwheat (50g)

The Salsa:

- Tomato (1 @ 130g)
- Capers (1 tbsp.)
- Bird's eye chili (1)
- Parsley (5g)
- Juice (1/4 of 1 lemon)

Method for Preparation:

1. Chop the kale and onion. Finely chop the tomatoes, capers, and parsley.
2. To make the salsa, add the tomato with juices and mix with the chili, capers, lemon juice, and parsley.
3. Heat the oven to 425° Fahrenheit/220°Celsius/gas 7.
4. Prepare the marinade for the chicken breast in the lemon juice, one teaspoon of the turmeric, and a portion of oil. Marinate it for five to ten minutes.
5. Warm an oven-proof skillet until hot, and add the chicken. Fry it for a minute or so on each side.
6. Place the pan into the heated oven for eight to ten minutes.
7. Transfer the pan to the countertop. Place a layer of foil over the top of the pan and wait for about five minutes before serving.
8. In the meantime, prepare the kale in a steamer for five minutes.
9. Sauté the ginger and onions in oil until softened. Fold in the steamed kale and stir fry the mixture for one more minute.
10. Prepare the buckwheat per the package directions with the rest of the turmeric. When it's ready, serve alongside the vegetables, chicken, and salsa.

Day 16: 1 Green Juice & 3 Meals - 1521 Calories

Daily Juice: Green Apple & Kiwi Juice: 547

Time Required: 5-8 minutes

Servings: 1
Nutritional Calories: 547

Ingredients Needed:
- Green apple (1)
- Kiwis (2)
- Celery stalk (1)
- Organic honey (.5 tbsp.)
- A pinch of pink Himalayan salt (1 pinch)
- Lime (half of 1)
- Turmeric (.5 tsp.)

Method for Preparation:
1. Chop the kiwis, celery, and apple.
2. Toss all of the components into a blender.
3. Mix it thoroughly and pour it into a cold glass.

Meal 1: Blueberry Muffins: 136
Time Required: 35-40 minutes
Servings: 8
Nutritional Calories: 136

Ingredients Needed:
- Buckwheat flour (1 cup)
- Arrowroot starch (.25 cup)
- Baking powder (1.5 tsp.)
- Sea salt (.25 tsp.)
- Eggs (2)
- Unsweetened almond milk (.5 cup)
- Melted coconut oil (2 tbsp.)
- Blueberries (1 cup - fresh)
- Maple syrup (2-3 tbsp.)

Method for Preparation:
1. Warm the oven to reach 350° Fahrenheit/177°Celsius. Prepare eight wells in a muffin tin.
2. Whisk the dry fixings (flour, baking powder, salt, and cornstarch).
3. In another dish, vigorously beat the eggs, oil, syrup, and milk.
4. Fold in the dry components until combined and add the berries.
5. Pour the mixture into the prepared cups.

6. Set the timer and bake for 25 minutes. Test for doneness using a toothpick. Poke the centers (it's ready when the pick is clean when removed).
7. Wait about ten minutes after you place the muffin tin on a wire rack before serving.

Meal 2: Prawn Arrabbiata: 733

Time Required: 1 hour 10 minutes
Servings: 1
Nutritional Calories: 733
Ingredients Needed:

- King Prawns - raw or cooked (125-150g)
- Buckwheat pasta (65 g)
- Olive oil (1 tbsp.)

The Sauce:

- Red onion (40g)
- Garlic (1 clove)
- Celery (30g)
- Dried mixed herbs (1 tsp.)
- Bird's eye chili (1)
- Olive oil (1 tsp.)
- Optional: White wine (2 tbsp.)
- Tinned chopped tomatoes (400g)
- Chopped parsley (1 tbsp.)

Method for Preparation:

1. Finely dice the onion, garlic, celery, parsley, and chili.
2. Sauté the garlic, dried herbs, onion, celery, and chili in the oil using the med-low temperature setting for one to two minutes. Adjust the temperature setting to medium. Pour in the wine and allow the mixture to simmer for one minute. Dump the tomatoes into the pan and continue to simmer using the med-low temperature setting (20-30 min.). Add a little water as needed for thinning.
3. Meanwhile, add water to a pan. Prepare the pasta, following the instructions on the package. Once it's cooked al dente, drain, and toss with the oil. Leave it in the pan until needed.
4. Add the raw prawns to the sauce and cook for about three to four minutes, until they're opaque/pink. Garnish using the parsley and serve.

Meal 3: Arugula & Berries Salad: 105
Time Required: 15 minutes
Servings: 4
Nutritional Calories: 105

Ingredients Needed:
- Fresh Berries: (.5 cup of each)
- Raspberries
- Blueberries
- Blackberries
- Strawberries (1 cup)
- Fresh arugula (6 cups)
- Olive oil (2 tbsp.)
- Ground black pepper & salt (as desired)

Method for Preparation:
1. Remove the hulls from the strawberries and slice. Toss with the rest of the fixings.
2. Serve in four bowls right away to preserve its nutrients.

Day 17: 1 Green Juice & 3 Meals - 1527 Calories

Meal 1: Sirtfood Scrambled Eggs: 224
Time Required: 35-40 minutes
Servings: 1
Nutritional Calories: 224

Ingredients Needed:
- Olive oil (1 tsp.)
- Red onion (20g/.75 oz.)
- Bird's eye chili (half of 1)
- Medium eggs (3)
- Milk (1.7 fl. oz./50 ml)
- Parsley (5g)
- Ground turmeric (1 tsp.)

Method for Preparation:
1. Finely chop the chili, parsley, and onion.
2. Warm the oil in a skillet using the high-temperature setting.

3. Toss in the chili and onion to sauté for two to three minutes.
4. Whisk the eggs, milk, turmeric, and parsley.
5. Dump the egg mixture into the skillet. Reduce the setting to the medium-temperature. Simmer for three to five minutes, scrambling with a spatula or spoon. Serve right away.

Meal 2: Coronation Chicken Salad: 831

Time Required: 5 minutes
Servings: 1
Nutritional Calories: 831

Ingredients Needed:

- Natural yogurt (75 g)
- Juice of ¼ of a lemon
- Ground turmeric (1 tsp.)
- Coriander (1 tsp.)
- Mild curry powder (.5 tsp.)
- Cooked chicken breast (100g)
- Walnut halves (6)
- Medjool date (1)
- Red onion (20g)
- Bird's eye chili (1)
- To Serve: Rocket/arugula (40g)

Method for Preparation:

1. Chop/dice the coriander, onion, walnut, and date. Slice the chicken into bite-sized chunks.
2. Mix the yogurt with the lemon juice, coriander, and spices in a mixing container.
3. Fold in the rest of the fixings and serve on a bed of the arugula.

Meal 3: Buckwheat Pasta Salad: 440

Time Required: 55 minutes
Servings: 2
Nutritional Calories: 440

Ingredients Needed:

- Buckwheat pasta (50g/1 5/8 oz.)
- Rocket (1 large handful)
- Cherry tomatoes (8)
- Avocado (half of 1)
- Olives (10)
- Olive oil (1 tbsp.)
- Basil leaves (1 small handful)
- To Garnish: Pine nuts (20g/.75 oz.)

Method for Preparation:

1. Slice the tomatoes into halves. Dice the avocado.
2. Toss each of the fixings into a salad dish. Portion the salad into two bowls.
3. Scatter the nuts on top and serve.

Daily Juice: Celery Juice: 32
Time Required: 10 minutes
Servings: 2
Nutritional Calories: 32

Ingredients Needed:

- Celery stalks with leaves (8)
- Fresh ginger (2 tbsp.)
- Lemon (1)
- Filtered water (.5 cup)
- Salt (1 pinch)

Method for Preparation:

1. Peel the lemon and ginger.
2. Toss each of the fixings into a blender and thoroughly puree until incorporated.
3. Strain the juice using a mesh strainer.
4. Serve in two glasses right away.

Day 18: 1 Green Juice & 3 Meals -1473 Calories

Daily Juice: Orange & Kale Juice: 315
Time Required: 10 minutes

Servings: 2
Nutritional Calories: 315

Ingredients Needed:

- Oranges (5 large)
- Fresh kale (2)

Method for Preparation:

1. Peel and break the orange into sections. Rinse the kale.
2. Add all of the fixings to a juicer and extract it accordingly.
3. Serve in two glasses when it's ready.

Meal 1: Buckwheat Porridge: 358
Time Required: 25 minutes
Servings: 2
Nutritional Calories: 358

Ingredients Needed:

- Water (1 cup)
- Buckwheat (1 cup)
- Almond milk - unsweetened (1 cup)
- Cinnamon (.5 tsp.)
- Vanilla extract (.5 tsp.)
- Fresh blueberries (.25 cup)
- Raw honey (1-2 tbsp.)

Method for Preparation:

1. Rinse the buckwheat and blueberries.
2. Prepare a saucepan using the medium-high temperature setting with all of the fixings except for the berries and honey. Wait for it to boil and switch the temperature to low.
3. Set the pan aside with a lid on it for about five minutes.
4. When ready, fluff the mixture, garnish with the berries, and serve.

Meal 2: Chili Con Carne: 346
Time Required: 2 hours 25-30 minutes
Servings: 4
Nutritional Calories: 346

Ingredients Needed:

- Red onion (1)
- Garlic cloves (3)
- Bird's eye chilies (2)
- Olive oil (1 tbsp.)
- Lean minced beef - 5 percent fat (400g)
- Red wine (150ml)
- Red pepper (1)
- Tomato purée (1 tbsp.)
- Chopped tomatoes (2 cans/400g each)
- Turmeric (1 tbsp.)
- Cocoa powder (1 tbsp.)
- Cumin (1 tbsp.)
- Kidney beans (150g - tinned)
- Beef stock (300ml)
- Coriander (5g)
- Parsley (5g)
- Buckwheat (160g)

Method for Preparation:

1. Core and remove the seeds from the red pepper and chop it into bite-sized pieces. Finely chop the parsley, coriander, onion, garlic, and chiles.
2. Cook the garlic, onion, and chili in the oil using a medium-temperature setting for two to three minutes, adding the spices to cook for a minute.
3. Fold in the minced beef and brown using the high heat temperature setting. Pour in the red wine and wait for it to bubble to reduce it by about half.
4. Add the tomatoes, red pepper, tomato purée, cocoa, kidney beans, and stock. Simmer them for about one hour.
5. Just before serving, stir in the chopped herbs.
6. Meanwhile, prepare the buckwheat per the package guidelines.
7. Serve with a smile!

Meal 2: Side Dish: Cucumber Salad With Coriander & Lime: 57

Time Required: 15 minutes

Servings: 2

Nutritional Calories: 57

Ingredients Needed:

- Red onion (1)
- Cucumber (2)
- Lime juice (2 limes)
- Fresh coriander (2 tbsp.)

Method for Preparation:

1. Thinly slice the cucumber and slice the onion into rings. Finely chop the coriander.
2. Toss the rings of onion into a mixing container, fill it with water, and about ½ tablespoon of salt.
3. When ready to use, dump them into a colander and rinse them thoroughly.
4. Toss everything together in a salad bowl, mixing well with salt.
5. Cover the dish and store to use for up to two or three days.

Meal 3: Baked Salmon Salad With Creamy Mint Dressing: 340

Time Required: 20 minutes
Servings: 1
Nutritional Calories: 340
Ingredients Needed:

- Salmon fillet (1 @ 130g)
- Young spinach leaves (40g)
- Mixed salad leaves (40g)
- Cucumber (5cm piece/50g)
- Radishes (2)
- Spring onions (2)
- Parsley (1 small handful/10g)

The Dressing:

- Natural yogurt (1 tbsp.)
- Mayonnaise - low-fat (1 tsp.)
- Rice vinegar (1 tbsp.)
- Mint (2 leaves)
- Freshly ground black pepper & salt (as desired)

Method for Preparation:

1. Thinly slice the radish. Chop the parsley and mint. Trim and slice the cucumber and spring into chunks.
2. Warm the oven to 200°Celcius/392° Fahrenheit (180°Celcius/356°

Fahrenheit fan/Gas @ 6).
3. Arrange the salmon fillet on a baking sheet with the skin side down. Bake it until just cooked through (16-18 min.). Remove the salmon from the skin after it has been cooked. Set it aside.
4. Combine the yogurt, mayo, vinegar, salt, pepper, and mint leaves. Wait for at least five minutes before serving it.
5. First, add the spinach on a serving plate with the onions, cucumber, radishes, and parsley.
6. Flake the prepared salmon over the salad with a spritz of dressing.
7. **Note:** Enjoy it hot or cold.

Meal 3: Cucumber Salad With Coriander & Lime: 57
Time Required: 15 minutes
Servings: 2
Nutritional Calories: 57

Ingredients Needed:
- Red onion (1)
- Cucumber (2)
- Lime juice (2 limes)
- Fresh coriander (2 tbsp.)

Method for Preparation:
1. Thinly slice the cucumber and slice the onion into rings. Finely chop the coriander.
2. Toss the rings of onion into a mixing container, fill it with water, and about ½ tablespoon of salt.
3. When ready to use, dump them into a colander and rinse them thoroughly.
4. Toss everything together in a salad bowl, mixing well with salt.
5. Cover the dish and store to use for up to two or three days.

Day 19: 1 Green Juice & 3 Meals - 1503 Calories

Daily Juice: Apple & Cucumber Juice: 230
Time Required: 10-12 minutes
Servings: 2

Nutritional Calories: 230

Ingredients Needed:

- Large apples (3)
- Cucumbers (2 large)
- Celery (4 stalks)
- Fresh ginger (1-inch/2.5cm piece)
- Lemon (1)

Method for Preparation:

1. Core and slice the apples and cucumbers. Peel the lemon and ginger.
2. Add each of the fixings into a juicer and extract the juice according to the manufacturer's directions.
3. Pour it into two chilled glasses to serve immediately.

Meal 1: Salmon & Kale Omelet: 210
Time Required: 17-20 minutes
Servings: 4
Nutritional Calories: 210

Ingredients Needed:

- Eggs (6)
- Unsweetened almond milk (2 tbsp.)
- Black pepper & salt (to your liking)
- Olive oil (2 tbsp.)
- Fresh kale (2 cups)
- Smoked salmon (4 oz.)
- Scallions (4)

Method for Preparation:

1. Prepare a wok using medium heat to warm the oil.
2. Trim the tough ribs off and chop the kale. Chop the salmon and kale into chunks. Finely chop the scallions.
3. Whisk the milk, salt, pepper, and eggs.
4. Dump the eggs into the wok and simmer them for about 30 seconds (no stirring).
5. Sprinkle the scallions, kale, and salmon over the eggs. Adjust the temperature setting to low.
6. Cover the wok using a lid and simmer for about four to five minutes.
7. Uncover the wok and simmer one additional minute before serving.

Meal 2: Lamb - Butternut Squash, & Date Tagine: 566
Time Required: 1.5 hours
Servings: 4
Nutritional Calories: 566

Ingredients Needed:

- Olive oil (2 tbsp.)
- Red onion (1)
- Ginger (2cm)
- Garlic (3 cloves)
- Chilli flakes (1 tsp./to taste)
- Cumin seeds (2 tsp.)
- Cinnamon (1 stick)
- Ground turmeric (2 tsp.)
- Lamb neck fillet (800g)
- Salt (.5 tsp.)
- Medjool dates - pitted (100g)
- Diced tomatoes (2 cups/ 400 g can + half a can of water)
- Chickpeas (400g tin)
- Butternut squash (500g)
- Fresh coriander (2 tbsp + more for the garnish)
- To Serve: Buckwheat/rice/couscous/flatbread

Method for Preparation:

1. Warm the oven at 284° Fahrenheit/140 °Celsius
2. Rinse and drain the chickpeas. Slice the onion. Mince the garlic and ginger. Chop the dates, lamb (2cm chunks), and squash (1cm cubes).
3. Warm two tablespoons of olive oil into a cast-iron casserole dish or sizeable oven-proof saucepan.
4. Sauté the sliced onion with the lid on until the onions are softened but not brown (5 min.).
5. Toss in the chili, ginger, garlic, cinnamon, turmeric, and cumin. Sauté for one more minute with the lid off. Add a sprinkle of water as needed.
6. Fold in the chunks of lamb, stirring thoroughly.
7. Mix in the dates, salt, and tomatoes, with half a can of water (100-200ml).
8. Wait for the tagine to boil - with a lid on - and cook for 1 ¼ hour.
9. About ½ an hour before the end of the cooking cycle, mix in the chickpeas and chopped butternut squash. Stir thoroughly, top it, and return to the oven for the final half-hour.
10. When the tagine is ready, transfer it to the countertop and mix in the chopped coriander.

11. Garnish as desired to serve.

Meal 3: Turmeric Chicken & Kale Salad & Lime Dressing: 393

Time Required: ½ hour
Servings: 2
Nutritional Calories: 393

Ingredients Needed:

- Ghee (1 tsp.) or Coconut oil (1 tbsp.)
- Brown onion (half of 1 medium)
- Chicken thighs (250-300g/9 oz.)
- Large garlic clove (1)
- Turmeric powder (1 tsp.)
- Lime zest (1 tsp.)
- Juice of ½ lime
- Salt + pepper (.5 tsp. of each)

The Salad:

- Broccoli florets (2 cups) or Broccolini (6 stalks)
- Pumpkin seeds - pepitas (2 tbsp.)
- Kale leaves (3 large)
- Avocado (half of 1)
- Coriander & Parsley leaves (1 freshly chopped handful of each)

The Dressing:

- Lime juice (3 tbsp.)
- Garlic clove (1 small)
- Olive oil (3 tbsp.) *or* Avocado oil (1 tbsp.) + Olive oil (2 tbsp.)
- Raw honey (1 tsp.)
- Whole grain - Dijon mustard (.5 tsp.)
- Black pepper & sea salt (.5 tsp. each)

Method for Preparation:

1. Finely dice the onion, garlic, and chicken. Remove the stems from the kale. Chop the parsley, kale, and coriander. Slice the avocado.
2. Warm the ghee/oil in a skillet using the med-high temperature setting.
3. Toss in the onion and sauté on medium heat for four to five minutes.
4. Add the chicken mince and garlic. Sauté them for two to three minutes using the med-high temperature, breaking it apart during the process.

5. Add the lime zest, turmeric, lime juice, pepper, and salt. Cook, often stirring for another three to four minutes.
6. Meanwhile, prepare a saucepan with water and cook the broccolini for two minutes. Rinse under cold tap water and slice them into three to four pieces each.
7. Toss the pumpkin seeds into the skillet (from the chicken) and toast using a medium-temperature setting for about two minutes. Sprinkle a bit of salt. Set it aside for now.
8. Place the chopped kale in a salad mixing container and garnish using the dressing. Toss and massage the kale with the dressing (using your hands).
9. Lastly, toss the cooked chicken, pumpkin seeds, fresh herbs, broccolini, and avocado slices.

Meal 3: Snack: Chocolate Bites: 104

Time Required: 15 minutes
Servings: 15
Nutritional Calories: 104

Ingredients Needed:

- Pitted dates (1 cup)
- Rolled oats - gluten-free preferred (2/3 cup)
- Chia seeds (1 tbsp.)
- Dark chocolate - unsweetened (.25 cup)
- Almond butter (3 tbsp.)
- Cacao powder (.5 cup)

Method for Preparation:

1. Prepare a baking tray using a layer of parchment paper.
2. Toss the dates into a food processor, pulsing until finely chopped.
3. Toss in the remainder of the fixings (omit the cacao), pulsing until it's just combined.
4. Prepare the mixture into one-inch balls and roll them in a bowl with the cacao powder. Place them on the baking tray.
5. Pop the bites into the freezer for about 15 minutes until they are set before serving.

Day 20: 1 Green Juice & 3 Meals - 1479 Calories

Daily Juice: Kale & Fruit Juice: 293

Time Required: 10 minutes
Servings: 2
Nutritional Calories: 293

Ingredients Needed:

- Green apples (2 large)
- Fresh kale (3 cups)
- Large pears (2)
- Celery (3 stalks)
- Lemon (1)

Method for Preparation:

1. Peel the lemon. Remove the core and slice the pears and apples.
2. Toss each of the components into a juicer.
3. Remove the juice and pour it into two chilled glasses to serve.

Meal 1: Kale & Mushroom Frittata: 151
Time Required: 45 minutes
Servings: 5
Nutritional Calories: 151
Ingredients Needed:

- Eggs (8)
- Unsweetened almond milk (.5 cup)
- Olive oil (1 tbsp.)
- Salt and freshly cracked black pepper (as desired)
- Onion (1)
- Garlic (1 clove)
- Mushrooms (1 cup)
- Fresh kale (1.5 cups)

Method for Preparation:

1. Chop/mince the mushrooms, garlic, and onion. Remove the ribs from the kale and chop.
2. Set the oven at 350° Fahrenheit/177° Celsius.
3. Whisk the eggs, pepper, salt, and milk.
4. Heat oil in a wok using the medium-temperature setting.
5. Sauté the garlic and onion for about three to four minutes.

6. Toss in the mushrooms, pepper, and salt. Sauté them for about eight to ten minutes.
7. Fold in the kale and simmer for another five minutes. Fold in the egg mixture and simmer it for about four minutes (do not stir).
8. Add them to the skillet in the oven to bake for 12 to 15 minutes.
9. Wait for it to cool for about five minutes before slicing to serve.

Meal 2: Asian King Prawn Stir-Fry & Buckwheat Noodles: 838
Time Required: 55 minutes
Servings: 2
Nutritional Calories:

Ingredients Needed:
- Raw king prawns (150g)
- Tamari or soy sauce (2 tbsp.)
- Soba/buckwheat noodles (75 g)
- Olive oil (2 tbsp.)
- Garlic (1 clove)
- Bird's eye chili (1)
- Fresh ginger (1 tsp.)
- Red onion (20g)
- Celery (40g)
- Green beans (75g)
- Kale (50g)
- Chicken stock (100 ml)
- Lovage/celery leaves (5g)

Method for Preparation:
1. Devein and shell the prawns. Finely chop the garlic, chili, and ginger. Trim and slice the celery and onion. Roughly chop the green beans and kale.
2. Warm a skillet using the high-temperature setting. Prepare the prawns in one teaspoon each of the tamari and oil for two to three minutes. At that time, place the prawns on a plate. Wipe the pan clean using a paper towel.
3. Prepare a pot of boiling water to cook the noodles for five to eight minutes or as indicated on the package. Pour them into a colander to drain and place to the side for now.
4. Meanwhile, fry the chili, celery, ginger, garlic, beans, red onion, and kale in the rest of the oil using the med-high temperature setting for

two to three minutes.

5. Pour in the stock and wait for it to boil. Simmer for about one to two minutes or until the veggies are cooked - yet still crunchy.
6. Mix in the noodles, prawns, and celery leaves to the pan. Reheat and transfer them from the heat to serve.

Meal 3: Chicken With Broccoli & Mushrooms: 197

Time Required: 40 minutes
Servings: 6
Nutritional Calories: 197

Ingredients Needed:

- Olive oil (3 tbsp.)
- Breasts of chicken (1 lb.)
- Medium onion (1)
- Garlic cloves (6)
- Mushrooms (2 cups)
- Small broccoli florets (16 oz.)
- Water (.25 cup)
- Ground black pepper and salt (to your liking)

Method for Preparation:

1. Do the prep. Remove the skin and bones from the chicken and chop it. Mince the garlic and chop the onions. Slice the mushrooms.
2. Warm the oil in a large wok using the medium temperature setting.
3. Toss in the chicken and sauté them for about four to five minutes.
4. Drain the chicken on a platter when done.
5. Toss the onion into the wok and sauté them for about four to five minutes. Stir in the mushrooms and continue to sauté them for four to five more minutes.
6. Stir in the chicken, water, salt, pepper, broccoli, and cook with a lid on the pot for eight to ten minutes, stirring intermittently.
7. Take the pan from the burner and serve piping hot.

Day 21: 1 Green Juice & 3 Meals - 1482 Calories

Daily Juice: Kale - Carrot & Grapefruit Juice: 232
Time Required: 10 minutes
Servings: 2
Nutritional Calories: 232

Ingredients Needed:
- Granny Smith apple (2 large)
- Fresh kale (3 cups)
- Fresh juice (1 tsp./1 lemon)
- Grapefruit (2 medium)
- Carrots (2)

Method for Preparation:
1. Peel the carrots and grapefruit. Slice and core the apple. Chop the carrots. Section the grapefruit, and squeeze the juice.
2. Toss the prepared foods into the juicer.
3. Extract the juice and pour it into two cold glasses to serve.

Meal 1: Date Walnut Porridge: 66
Time Required: 1.5 hours
Servings: 2
Nutritional Calories: 66

Ingredients Needed:
- Milk/Dairy of choice (200 ml/6.5 fl.oz.)
- Chopped Medjool date (1)
- Buckwheat chips (1.25 oz./35g)

Step 2:
- Pecan spread/4 halved pecans (1 tsp.)
- Hulled strawberries (1- 5/8 oz./20g)

Method for Preparation:
1. Combine each of the fixings in a dish and warm until it reaches the desired consistency.
2. Mix in the pecans and top with the berries to serve.

Meal 2: Turmeric Baked Salmon: 654
Time Required: 25-30 minutes

Servings: 1
Nutritional Calories: 654

Ingredients Needed:

- Skinned salmon (125-150g)
- Ground turmeric (1 tsp.)
- Olive oil (1 tsp.)
- Juice (¼ to ½ of 1 lemon)

The Celery:

- Tinned green lentils (60g)
- Olive oil (1 tsp.)
- Red onion (40g)
- Garlic (1 clove)
- Fresh ginger (1 cm)
- Bird's eye chili (1)
- Celery (150g/2cm lengths)
- Mild curry powder (1 tsp.)
- Tomato (130g/8 wedges)
- Chicken or vegetable stock (100 ml)
- Chopped parsley (1 tbsp.)

Method for Preparation:

1. Dice the chili, onion, garlic, and ginger.
2. Heat the oven to 392° Fahrenheit/200° Celsius or at the gas mark 6.
3. Warm a skillet using the med-low temperature setting, add the oil, chili, onion, ginger, garlic, and celery. Fry gently for two to three minutes or until softened - not colored. Mix in the curry powder and sauté it for another minute.
4. Pour in the tomatoes, lentils, and stock. Simmer gently for ten minutes. Adjust the cooking time, depending on the crispiness desired.
5. Mix the lemon juice with the oil and turmeric. Rub the mixture over the salmon.
6. Arrange the prepared salmon on a baking tray. Cook it for eight to ten minutes.
7. Garnish it using the parsley and celery. Serve with the salmon.

Meal 3: Bunless Burger With The Trimmings: 530

Time Required: 45 minutes
Servings: 1
Nutritional Calories: 530

Ingredients Needed:

- Lean minced beef - 5% fat (125g)
- Red onion (15g)
- Parsley (1 tsp.)
- Olive oil (1 tsp.)
- Sweet potatoes (150g)
- Dried rosemary (1 tsp.)
- Garlic clove (1 unpeeled)
- Cheddar cheese - sliced or grated (10g)
- Red onion (150g)
- Tomato (30g)
- Rocket (10g)
- Optional: Gherkin (1)

Method for Preparation:

1. Finely chop the garlic, parsley, and onion. Slice the tomato and onions into rings.
2. Heat the oven to 420° Fahrenheit/220° Celsius/gas 7.
3. Peel and cut the sweet potato into 1cm thick chips. Toss them with the rosemary, oil, and garlic clove. Arrange them on a baking tray and roast until crispy (30 min.).
4. Mix the onion and parsley with the minced beef and shape them into patties.
5. Warm a skillet using the medium temperature setting to warm the oil.
6. Place the burger on one side of the pan, and the onion rings on the other.
7. Cook the burger for six minutes per side, ensuring it's thoroughly cooked as desired. Fry the onion rings until they are crispy.
8. Prepare the burger with the cheese and onion.
9. Put them on a baking sheet and place them in the hot oven for a minute to melt the cheese.
10. Remove and top and add the tomato, rocket, and gherkin. Serve with the fries.

At this point, you are on your own. Research has you to this point but needs more time to pursue the plan further. How are your results?

At the end of the 21 days, you can repeat the phases of the plan as often as desired. You should continue consuming the 'sirtfoods' in your diet as a snack or other meals. Using this process will allow you to change your lifestyle.

You should have a good idea of how to manage the diet plan the next time you decide you want to quickly drop a few pounds. Now, it's time to stick with the foods and maintain your newly acquired weight loss. I will provide you with one more week in this segment.

Chapter 6: On Your Own-Week 4

It is suggested to continue drinking one green juice each day!

Day 22

Daily Juice: Apple-Cherry Juice
Time Required: 10 minutes
Servings: 2
Nutritional Calories: 240

Ingredients Needed:

- Green apples (4 large)
- Celery stalks (4)
- Lemon (1)

Method for Preparation:

1. Peel, core, and slice the apples. Peel the lemon.
2. Toss the fixings into a juicer.
3. When it's ready, pour into two glasses and serve.

Meal 1: Buckwheat Porridge
Time Required: 25 minutes
Servings: 2

Nutritional Calories: 358

Ingredients Needed:

- Water (1 cup)
- Buckwheat (1 cup)
- Almond milk - unsweetened (1 cup)
- Cinnamon (.5 tsp.)
- Vanilla extract (.5 tsp.)
- Fresh blueberries (.25 cup)
- Raw honey (1-2 tbsp.)

Method for Preparation:

1. Rinse the buckwheat and blueberries.
2. Prepare a saucepan using the medium-high temperature setting with all of the fixings except for the berries and honey. Wait for it to boil and switch the temperature to low.
3. Set the pan aside with a lid on it for about five minutes.
4. When ready, fluff the mixture, garnish with the berries, and serve.

Meal 2: Bunless Burger With The Trimmings

Time Required: 45 minutes
Servings: 1
Nutritional Calories: 530

Ingredients Needed:

- Lean minced beef - 5% fat (125g)
- Red onion (15g)
- Parsley (1 tsp.)
- Olive oil (1 tsp.)
- Sweet potatoes (150g)
- Dried rosemary (1 tsp.)
- Garlic clove (1 unpeeled)
- Cheddar cheese - sliced or grated (10g)
- Red onion (150g)
- Tomato (30g)
- Rocket (10g)
- Optional: Gherkin (1)

Method for Preparation:

1. Finely chop the garlic, parsley, and onion. Slice the tomato and onions into rings.
2. Heat the oven to 420° Fahrenheit/220° Celsius/gas 7.
3. Peel and slice the potato into chips (1 cm thickness). Toss them with the rosemary, oil, and garlic clove. Arrange them on a baking tray and roast until crispy (30 min.).
4. Mix the onion and parsley with the minced beef and shape them into patties.
5. Warm a skillet using the medium-temperature setting to warm the oil.
6. Place the burger on one side of the pan, and the onion rings on the other.
7. Cook the burger for six minutes per side, ensuring it's thoroughly cooked as desired. Fry the onion rings until they are crispy.
8. Prepare the burger with the cheese and onion.
9. Put them on a baking tray and pop them into the hot oven for a minute to melt the cheese.
10. Remove and top and add the tomato, rocket, and gherkin.

Meal 3: Chicken - Kale & Sprout Stir-Fry

Time Required: ½ hour
Servings: 2
Nutritional Calories: 390

Ingredients Needed:

- Soba noodles (100g)
- Shredded curly kale (100g)
- Sesame oil (2 tsp.)
- Lean chicken breasts (2 - in strips - no skin)
- Fresh ginger (25g piece)
- Red pepper (1)
- Brussels sprouts (1 handful/as desired)
- Soy sauce - l.s. (1 tbsp.)
- Rice wine vinegar (2 tbsp.)
- Lime (1 - juiced & zested)

Method for Preparation:

1. Peel and slice the ginger into matchsticks. Cut the sprouts into quarters. Deseed the pepper and slice it thin. Zest and juice the lime. Cook the

noodles until they are al dente. Dump them into a colander to drain.

2. In the meantime, warm a large skillet/wok, and add the kale with a good splash of water. Simmer for one to two minutes until wilted. Remove and run the kale under cold - running water to keep the color.
3. Add half the oil and fry the chicken strips until browned. Transfer them to a platter and set aside.
4. Warm the rest of the oil and fry the pepper, ginger, and sprouts until slightly softened. Place the chicken and kale in with them and add the noodles.
5. Mix in the soy, lime zest and juice, and rice wine with enough water to create a sauce that clings to the ingredients. Serve and enjoy it promptly for the best results.

Day 23

Daily Juice: Apple-Cucumber Juice
Time Required: 10-12 minutes
Servings: 2
Nutritional Calories: 230

Ingredients Needed:

- Large apples (3)
- Cucumbers (2 large)
- Celery (4 stalks)
- Fresh ginger (1-inch/2.5cm piece)
- Lemon (1)

Method for Preparation:

1. Core and slice the cucumbers and apples. Peel the ginger and lemon.
2. Add each of the ingredients into a juicer and extract the juice.
3. Pour it into two cold glasses and enjoy it immediately.

Meal 1: Kale & Mushroom Frittata
Time Required: 45 minutes
Servings: 5
Nutritional Calories: 151
Ingredients Needed:

- Eggs (8)
- Unsweetened almond milk (.5 cup)
- Olive oil (1 tbsp.)
- Salt and freshly cracked black pepper (as desired)
- Onion (1)
- Garlic (1 clove)
- Mushrooms (1 cup)
- Fresh kale (1.5 cups)

Method for Preparation:

1. Chop/mince the mushrooms, garlic, and onion. Remove the ribs from the kale and chop.
2. Set the oven at 350° Fahrenheit/177° Celsius.
3. Whisk the eggs, pepper, salt, and milk.
4. Heat oil in a wok using the medium-temperature setting.
5. Sauté the garlic and onion for about three to four minutes.
6. Toss in the mushrooms, pepper, and salt. Sauté them for about eight to ten minutes.
7. Fold in the kale and simmer for another five minutes. Fold in the egg mixture and simmer it for about four minutes (do not stir).
8. Add them to the skillet in the oven to bake for 12 to 15 minutes.
9. Wait for it to cool for about five minutes before slicing to serve.

Meal 2: South Indian Malabar Prawns

Time Required: 26-30 minutes
Servings: 4
Nutritional Calories: 171

Ingredients Needed:

- King prawns (400g raw)
- Kashmiri chili powder (3-4 tsp.)
- Turmeric (2 tsp.)
- Lemon juice (4 tsp. + a squeeze)
- Ginger (40g)
- Vegetable oil (1 tbsp.)
- Curry leaves (4)
- Green chiles (2-4)
- Onion (1)
- Black pepper (1 tsp.)
- Fresh coconut (40g)

- Coriander leaves (half of 1 small bunch)

Method for Preparation:

1. Slice the chiles into halves and remove the seeds. Peel and grate half of the ginger, and slice the other half into matchsticks. Finely slice the onion and grate the coconut.
2. Rinse the prawns in cold water and pat dry. Toss them with the turmeric, chili, lemon juice, and grated ginger. Wait a few minutes for the fixings to combine their flavors.
3. Warm the oil in a skillet and toss in the chili, curry leaves, sliced ginger, and onion. Cook the mixture until translucent (10 min.) Add the black pepper.
4. Toss the prawns in with any marinade, and stir-fry until cooked (2 min.).
5. Season as desired and add a squeeze of lemon juice.
6. Garnish the prawns using the coconut and coriander leaves.

Meal 3: Asian Hot Pot
Time Required: 15 minutes
Servings: 2
Nutritional Calories: 185

Ingredients Needed:

- Tomato purée (1 tsp.)
- Star anise (1 crushed) or Ground anise (.25 tsp.)
- Parsley (small handful/10g)
- Coriander (10g/small handful)
- Lime juice (half of 1 lime)
- Chicken stock (500ml - fresh or /1 cube)
- Carrot (half of 1)
- Broccoli (50g)
- Beansprouts (50g)
- Raw tiger prawns (100g)
- Firm tofu (100g)
- Rice noodles (50g)
- Cooked water chestnuts (50g)
- Sushi ginger (20g)
- Good-quality miso paste (1 tbsp.)

Method for Preparation:

1. Prepare the noodles by following the packet instructions.

2. Drain the water chestnuts. Finely chop the ginger, parsley, and coriander. Chop the tofu. Peel and cut the carrots into matchsticks and the broccoli into florets.
3. Pour the tomato purée, star anise, parsley stalks, coriander stalks, lime juice, and chicken stock in a large saucepan and bring to a simmer for about ten minutes.
4. Toss in the broccoli, carrot, prawns, noodles, tofu, and water chestnuts.
5. Simmer gently until the prawns are cooked thoroughly. Transfer them from the heat and stir in the sushi ginger and miso paste.
6. Serve when ready. Sprinkle with the parsley and coriander leaves.

Day 24

Daily Juice: Grape & Melon Juice
Time Required: 3 minutes
Servings: 1
Nutritional Calories: 125

Ingredients Needed:

- Cucumber (half of 1)
- Spinach (30g baby leaves)
- Red seedless grapes (100g)
- Cantaloupe melon (100g)

Method for Preparation

1. Peel and deseed the melon of choice into chunks.
2. Peel (or not) the cucumber, remove the seeds and chop it. Remove the stalks from the spinach.
3. Combine each of the fixings in a juicer/blender and combine until it's smooth.

Meal 1: Shakshuka
Time Required: 45 minutes
Servings: 1
Nutritional Calories: 607
Ingredients Needed:

- Olive oil (1 tsp.)

- Red onion (40g)
- Garlic clove (1)
- Celery (30g)
- Bird's eye chili (1)
- Paprika (1 tsp.)
- Ground cumin (1 tsp.)
- Ground turmeric (1 tsp.)
- Tinned chopped tomatoes (400g)
- Kale (30g)
- Chopped parsley (1 tbsp.)
- Medium eggs (2)

Method for Preparation:

1. Finely chop the onion, clove, celery, and chili pepper. Remove the stems and roughly chop the kale and parsley.
2. Warm a deep-sided frying pan using the med-low temperature setting to warm the oil. Add and sauté the garlic, celery, onion, chili, and spices for one to two minutes.
3. Stir in the tomatoes, then leave the sauce to simmer gently for 20 minutes, occasionally stirring.
4. Fold in the kale and simmer for another five minutes. If the sauce is too thick, mix in a little water. When your sauce has a rich consistency, stir in the parsley.
5. Make two little wells in the sauce and crack each egg into them. Adjust the temperature to its lowest setting. Place a lid over the pan to cook. Leave the eggs to cook for 10–12 minutes, at which point the whites should be firm while the yolks are still runny. Cook for another 3–4 minutes if you prefer the yolks to be firm.
6. Serve immediately – ideally straight from the pan.

Meal 2: Chicken With Broccoli & Mushrooms

Time Required: 40-45 minutes
Servings: 6
Nutritional Calories: 197

Ingredients Needed:

- Olive oil (3 tbsp.)

- Breasts of chicken (1 lb.)
- Medium onion (1)
- Garlic cloves (6)
- Mushrooms (2 cups)
- Small broccoli florets (16 oz.)
- Water (.25 cup)
- Salt & freshly ground black pepper (as desired)

Method for Preparation:

1. Do the prep. Trim the bones and skin from the chicken and chop it. Mince the garlic and chop the onions. Slice the mushrooms.
2. Warm the oil in a large wok using the medium temperature setting.
3. Toss in the chicken and sauté them for about four to five minutes.
4. Drain the chicken on a platter when done.
5. Toss the onion into the wok and sauté them for about four to five minutes. Stir in the mushrooms and continue to sauté them for four to five more minutes.
6. Stir in the chicken, water, salt, pepper, broccoli, and cook with a lid on the pot for eight to ten minutes, stirring intermittently.
7. Take the pan from the burner and serve piping hot.

Meal 3: Turmeric Baked Salmon

Time Required: 25 minutes to ½ hour
Servings: 1
Nutritional Calories: 654

Ingredients Needed:

- Skinned salmon (125-150g)
- Ground turmeric (1 tsp.)
- Olive oil (1 tsp.)
- Juice (¼ to ½ of 1 lemon)

The Celery:

- Tinned green lentils (60g)
- Olive oil (1 tsp.)
- Red onion (40g)
- Garlic (1 clove)
- Fresh ginger (1 cm)
- Bird's eye chili (1)
- Celery (150g/2cm lengths)
- Mild curry powder (1 tsp.)
- Tomato (130g/8 wedges)

- Chicken or vegetable stock (100 ml)
- Chopped parsley (1 tbsp.)

Method for Preparation:

1. Dice the garlic, onion, chili, and ginger.
2. Heat the oven to 392° Fahrenheit/200° Celsius/gas mark @ 6.
3. Warm a skillet using the med-low temperature setting, add the oil, chili, onion, ginger, garlic, and celery. Fry gently for two to three minutes or until softened - not colored. Mix in the curry powder and sauté it for another minute.
4. Pour in the tomatoes, lentils, and stock. Simmer gently for ten minutes. Adjust the cooking time, depending on how crispy you like your celery.
5. Mix the oil with the lemon juice and turmeric; rub over the salmon.
6. Arrange the prepared salmon on a baking tray to cook for eight to ten minutes.
7. Garnish it using the parsley and celery. Serve with the salmon.

Day 25

Daily Juice: Broccoli - Apple & Orange Juice
Time Required: 10 minutes
Servings: 2
Nutritional Calories: 254

Ingredients Needed:

- Oranges (3 large)
- Broccoli (2 stalks)
- Fresh parsley (4 tbsp.)
- Sliced green apples (2 large)

Method for Preparation:

1. Use a sharp knife to remove the core from the apples. Chop the broccoli. Peel and section the oranges.
2. Toss all of the ingredients into a juicer and extract the juice.
3. Pour and serve in two ice-cold glasses to enjoy promptly.

Meal 1: Date Walnut Porridge
Time Required: 1 ½ hour

Servings: 2
Nutritional Calories: 66

Ingredients Needed:

- Milk/Dairy of choice (200 ml/6.5 fl.oz.)
- Chopped Medjool date (1)
- Buckwheat chips (1.25 oz./35g)

Step 2:

- Pecan spread/4 halved pecans (1 tsp.)
- Strawberries (20g or 1- 5/8 oz.)

Method for Preparation:

1. Chop the date and remove the hull from the berries.
2. Combine each of the fixings in a dish and warm until it reaches the desired consistency.
3. Mix in the pecans and top with the berries to serve.

Meal 2: Sirt Salmon Super Salad
Time Required: 10 minutes
Servings: 1
Nutritional Calories: 444

Ingredients Needed:

- Rocket (50g)
- Chicory leaves (50g)
- Smoked salmon slices (100g)
- Avocado (80g)
- Celery (40g)
- Red onion (20g)
- Walnuts (15g)
- Capers (1 tbsp.)
- Medjool date - pitted (1 large)
- Olive oil (1 tbsp.)
- Juice of ¼ lemon
- Parsley (10g)
- Lovage or celery leaves (10g)

Method for Preparation:

1. Chop the date, parsley, lovage, and walnuts, and slice the celery. Remove the stone, peel, and slice the avocado. Dice the onion. Arrange the salad leaves in a large salad dish.
2. Combine all of the fixings and serve over the leaves.

Meal 3: Bok Choy & Mushroom Stir-Fry

Time Required: 25 minutes
Servings: 4
Nutritional Calories: 77

Ingredients Needed:

- Olive oil (4 tsp.)
- Baby bok choy (1 lb.)
- Fresh ginger (1 tsp.)
- Mushrooms (5 oz.)
- Garlic cloves (2)
- Soy sauce (2 tbsp.)
- Red wine (2 tbsp.)
- Black pepper (to your liking)

Method for Preparation:

1. Mince the ginger and garlic. Slice the mushrooms and trim the bok choy base. Remove the outer leaves from the stalks - leaving the inner leaves attached.
2. Prepare a cast-iron skillet to warm the oil using the med-high temperature setting.
3. Toss in the garlic and ginger to sauté for about 60 seconds.
4. Add in the mushrooms to sauté for four to five minutes, stirring often.
5. Fold in the bok choy leaves and stalks. Simmer for about one minute, moving it around using tongs.
6. Stir in the soy sauce, wine, and pepper. Simmer for another two to three minutes, tossing intermittently, and serve it hot.

Day 26

Daily Juice: Green Apple & Kiwi Juice
Time Required: 5-9 minutes
Servings: 1
Nutritional Calories: 547

Ingredients Needed:
- Green apple (1)
- Kiwis (2)
- Celery stalk (1)
- Lime (half of 1)
- Organic honey (.5 tbsp.)
- A pinch of pink Himalayan salt (1 pinch)
- Turmeric (.5 tsp.)

Method for Preparation:
1. Roughly chop the celery, kiwis, and apple.
2. Toss each of the fixings into your blender.
3. Blend them thoroughly and pour them into an ice-cold glass.

Meal 1: Arugula & Berries Salad
Time Required: 15 minutes
Servings: 4
Nutritional Calories: 105

Ingredients Needed:
- Fresh arugula (6 cups)
- Fresh berries: (.5 cup each)
- Blueberries
- Raspberries
- Blackberries
- Strawberries (1 cup)
- Olive oil (2 tbsp.)
- Salt and freshly ground black pepper (as desired)

Method for Preparation:
1. Remove the hulls from the strawberries and slice. Toss with the rest of the fixings.
2. Serve in four bowls right away to preserve its nutrients.

Meal 2: Chili Con Carne
Time Required: 2.5 hours - varies
Servings: 4
Nutritional Calories: 346

Ingredients Needed:
- Coriander (5g)
- Parsley (5g)
- Buckwheat (160g)
- Bird's eye chilies (2)
- Red onion (1)
- Garlic cloves (3)
- Olive oil (1 tbsp.)
- Lean minced beef - 5 % fat (400g)
- Red wine (150ml)
- Red pepper (1)
- Tomato purée (1 tbsp.)
- Chopped tomatoes (2 cans/400g each)
- Cocoa powder (1 tbsp.)
- Turmeric (1 tbsp.)
- Cumin (1 tbsp.)
- Kidney beans (150g - tinned)
- Beef stock (300ml)

Method for Preparation:
1. Remove the core and seeds from the red pepper and chop it into bite-sized pieces. Finely chop the garlic, coriander, parsley, onion, and chiles.
2. Cook the garlic, onion, and chili in the oil using a medium-temperature setting for two to three minutes, adding the spices to cook for a minute.
3. Fold in the minced beef and brown using the high heat temperature setting. Pour in the red wine and wait for it to bubble to reduce it by about half.
4. Add the tomatoes, red pepper, tomato purée, cocoa, kidney beans, and

stock. Simmer them for about one hour.
5. Just before serving, stir in the chopped herbs.
6. Meanwhile, prepare the buckwheat per the package guidelines.
7. Serve with the chili.

Meal 3: Chicken - Veggies & Buckwheat Noodles
Time Required: 45 minutes
Servings: 2
Nutritional Calories: 463

Ingredients Needed:

- Broccoli florets (.5 cup)
- Fresh green beans (.5 cup)
- Buckwheat noodles (5 oz.)
- Fresh kale (1 cup)
- Coconut oil (1 tbsp.)
- Brown onion (1)
- Cubed chicken breast (6 oz.)
- Garlic (2 cloves)
- Soy sauce - low-sodium (3 tbsp.)

Method for Preparation:

1. Trim and slice the beans. Remove the tough kale ribs and chop them. Finely chop the cloves and onion. Cube the chicken.
2. Prepare a pan of boiling water. Toss in the green beans and broccoli to steam for four to five minutes.
3. Toss in the kale, and cook another one to two minutes.
4. Drain the veggies and place them in a container. Set them aside for now.
5. Prepare another pan with boiling salted water and cook the noodles for five minutes.
6. Drain and rinse the noodles.
7. Prepare a large wok with oil. Using medium heat, toss in and sauté the onion for two to three minutes. Fold in the cubed chicken and cook for another five to six minutes.
8. Mix in the soy sauce, garlic, and a splash of water. Simmer for two to three minutes, stirring often.
9. Stir in the veggies and noodles. Warm everything for one to two minutes, before serving with a garnish of sesame seeds.

Day 27

Daily Juice: Kale - Carrot & Grapefruit Juice
Time Required: 10 minutes
Servings: 2
Nutritional Calories: 232

Ingredients Needed:

- Carrots (2)
- Grapefruit (2 medium)
- Granny Smith apple (2 large)
- Fresh kale (3 cups)
- Fresh juice (1 tsp./1 lemon)

Method for Preparation:

1. Peel the carrots and grapefruit. Slice and core the apple. Chop the carrots. Section the grapefruit, and squeeze the juice.
2. Toss the prepared foods into the juicer.
3. Extract the juice and pour it into two cold glasses to serve.

Meal 1: Kale Scramble
Time Required: 16 minutes
Servings: 2
Nutritional Calories: 183

Ingredients Needed:

- Olive oil (2 tsp.)
- Eggs (4)
- Ground turmeric (1/8 tsp.)
- Black pepper & salt (as desired)
- Water (1 tbsp.)
- Kale (1 cup)

Method for Preparation:

1. Prep the fresh kale by removing the tough rib parts and chopping it apart to your liking.
2. Whisk the salt, pepper, turmeric, and eggs in a mixing container until they are foaming.
3. Heat a wok using the medium temperature setting.
4. Stir in the eggs and lower the setting to med-low. Cook them for one

to two minutes, continuing to scramble.
5. Fold in the kale and continue the process for three to four minutes, stirring often.
6. Serve and enjoy them immediately.

Meal 2: Baked Oriental Salmon & Broccoli Tray
Time Required: 30-35 minutes
Servings: 4
Nutritional Calories: 310

Ingredients Needed:
- Eggs (4)
- Ground turmeric (1/8 tsp.)
- Black pepper & salt (as desired)
- Water (1 tbsp.)
- Olive oil (2 tsp.)
- Kale (1 cup)

Method for Preparation:
1. Prepare the fresh kale by removing the tough rib parts and chopping it apart to your liking.
2. Whisk the salt, pepper, turmeric, and eggs in a mixing container until they are foaming.
3. Heat a wok using the medium temperature setting.
4. Stir in the eggs and lower the setting to med-low. Cook them for one to two minutes, continuing to scramble.
5. Fold in the kale and continue the process for three to four minutes, stirring often.
6. Serve and enjoy them promptly.

Meal 3: Chicken With Red Onion & Kale
Time Required: 30-35 minutes
Servings: 1
Nutritional Calories: 751

Ingredients Needed:
- Lemon juice (.25 tsp./to taste)

- Olive oil (1 tsp.)
- Turmeric powder - divided (2 tsp.)
- Chicken breast (120g)
- Tomatoes (130g)
- Bird's eye chili (1)
- Capers (1 tbsp.)
- Chopped parsley (5g)
- Kale (50g)
- Red onion (20g)
- Fresh ginger (1 tsp.)
- Buckwheat (50g)

Method for Preparation:

1. Warm the oven at 220° F/104° C.
2. Marinate the chicken for about ten minutes using ¼ teaspoon of juice, one teaspoon each of turmeric powder, and oil.
3. Slice the tomatoes into chunks and remove the inside. Sprinkle with the chili pepper, parsley, capers, turmeric (1 tsp.), lemon juice, and oil.
4. Drain the chicken. Use the high-temperature setting for cooking the chicken for one minute on each side. Pop it in the oven with a layer of foil over the top for about ten minutes.
5. Mince the kale and steam it in a saucepan for about five minutes.
6. Prepare a skillet with one teaspoon of oil, and sauté the freshly grated ginger and onion. Mix in the steamed cabbage for one minute.
7. Boil the buckwheat with the turmeric and drain. Serve it with the tomatoes, chicken, and chopped kale.

Day 28

Daily Juice: Lemony Green Juice

Time Required: 10 minutes
Servings: 2
Nutritional Calories: 196

Ingredients Needed:

- Lemon (1)
- Green apples (2 large)
- Fresh kale leaves (4 cups/67g)

- Fresh parsley leaves (4 tbsp./3.8g)
- Fresh ginger (1-inch piece/2.5cm/1 tbsp.)
- Filtered water (.5 cup/4 oz.)
- Salt (1 pinch)

Method for Preparation:

1. Remove the core and slice the apples. Peel the lemon and ginger.
2. Toss the fixings into a blender and mix until incorporated.
3. Remove and work it through a fine-mesh strainer to remove the juice.
4. Empty the juice into two chilled glasses and serve.

Meal 1: Strawberry Buckwheat Pancakes
Time Required: 45-50 minutes
Servings: 4
Nutritional Calories: 180

Ingredients Needed:

- Strawberries (3.5 oz.)
- Egg (1)
- Milk (8 fl. oz.)
- Buckwheat flour (3.5 oz.)
- Olive oil (1 tsp. + 1 tsp. for frying)
- Fresh juice (1 orange)

Method for Preparation:

1. Rinse and chop the berries.
2. Measure and add the milk and egg with one teaspoon of oil. Whisk the flour into the mixture and continue to mix it until creamy.
3. Wait for 15 minutes.
4. Warm oil in a pan and add ¼ of the batter or to the preferred size.
5. Add ¼ of the berries over the batter and cook for about two minutes per side.
6. Serve hot with a spritz of juice.
7. Tip: You could try blackberries or blueberries for a change of pace, but calculate the calories.

Meal 2: Beans & Kale Soup
Time Required: 45 minutes
Servings: 6
Nutritional Calories: 204

Ingredients Needed:

- Onions (2)
- Olive oil (2 tbsp.)
- Garlic (4 cloves)
- Kale (1 lb.)
- Cannellini beans (2 - 14 oz. cans)
- Water (6 cups)
- Black pepper & salt (as desired)

Method for Preparation:

1. Thoroughly rinse the beans in a colander and wait for them to drain. Chop the onions and garlic. Prep the kale (trimmed/ribs removed and chopped).
2. Warm the oil in a skillet using the medium temperature setting. Sauté the onions and garlic for about four to five minutes.
3. Toss in the kale and continue cooking for one to two more minutes.
4. Pour in the water, salt, pepper, and beans.
5. Once boiling, cook with the lid slightly ajar for about 15 to 20 minutes.
6. Serve them piping hot.

Meal 3: Turkey Escalope With Capers & Spiced Cauliflower Couscous

Time Required: 20 minutes
Servings: 1
Nutritional Calories: 454

Ingredients Needed:

- Cauliflower (150g)
- Garlic (1 clove)
- Red onion (40g)
- Bird's eye chili (1)
- Fresh ginger (1tsp.)
- Olive oil (2 tbsp.)
- Ground turmeric (2 tsp.)
- Sun-dried tomatoes (30g)
- Parsley (10g)
- Turkey escalope (150g)
- Dried sage (1 tsp.)
- Juice (½ lemon)
- Capers (1 tbsp.)

Method for Preparation:

1. Roughly chop and toss the cauliflower into a food processor.
2. Pulse it until it's finely chopped using two-second bursts to resemble couscous. Set the container aside.
3. Finely chop and sauté the ginger, onion, garlic, chili in one teaspoon of oil until softened. Mix in the cauliflower and turmeric to sauté for another minute. Transfer the pan from the burner and mix in the sun-dried tomatoes and half the parsley.
4. Coat the turkey escalope in the rest of the oil and sage. Cook it for five to six minutes, flipping it often.
5. When it's thoroughly cooked, stir in the remaining parsley, capers, lemon juice, and one tablespoon of water to make a sauce.
6. Enjoy it while it's piping hot.

Chapter 7: Sirtfood Breakfast Meal Options

Tomato Frittata
Time Required: 1 hour 15 minutes
Servings: 2
Nutritional Calories: 269

Ingredients Needed:

- Grated cheddar cheese (1- 5/8 oz. or 50g)
- Kalamata olives (2.25 oz./75g)
- Cherry tomatoes (8)
- Large eggs (4)
- Fresh basil & parsley (1 tbsp. each)
- Olive oil (1 tbsp.)

Method for Preparation:

1. Remove the pit and slice the olives and cherry tomatoes.
2. Chop the basil and parsley and mix it with the eggs, olives, cheese, and tomatoes.
3. Warm a skillet and heat the oil. Pour the egg mixture into the hot pan and cook for five to ten minutes until they're set.
4. Remove and place them under a broiler for about five minutes - until set.
5. Serve and enjoy them right away.

Sweet Breakfast Options

Apple Pancakes With Blackcurrant Compote
Time Required: 20-25 minutes
Servings: 4
Nutritional Calories: 337

Ingredients Needed:

- Porridge oats (75g)
- Plain flour (125g)
- Caster sugar (2 tbsp.)
- Salt (1 pinch)
- Baking powder (1 tsp.)
- Apples (2)
- Egg whites (2)
- Skim milk (300ml)
- Light olive oil (2 tsp.)

The Compote:

- Blackcurrants (120g)
- Caster sugar (2 tbsp.)
- Water (3 tbsp.)

Method for Preparation:

1. Peel, core, and chop the apple to bits. Rinse and remove the stalks from the blackcurrants.
2. Make the compote. Measure and add the blackcurrants, water, and sugar in a small saucepan. Once it's boiling, simmer for 10 to 15 minutes.
3. Measure and add the oats, salt, baking powder, flour, and sugar in a large mixing container. Fold in the small portions of the apple and whisk in the milk slowly until it's creamy smooth.
4. Briskly beat the whites of the eggs to form stiff peaks and fold the mix into the pancake batter. Transfer the batter to a jug.
5. Heat ½ teaspoon of oil in a skillet using the medium-high temperature setting.
6. Pour about ¼ of the batter into the skillet at a time, cooking until they are golden brown. Continue until you have four pancakes.
7. Serve the pancakes with a drizzle of the blackcurrant compote over the top.

Brunch Fruit Salad
Time Required: 10-15 minutes
Servings: 1
Nutritional Calories: 172

Ingredients Needed:

- Freshly brewed green tea (.5 cup)
- Honey (1 tsp.)
- Orange (1)
- Apple (1)
- Red seedless grapes (10)
- Blueberries (10)

Method for Preparation:

1. Slice the orange in half. Core and roughly chop the apple.
2. Prepare the tea and stir honey into half of a cup. After it is dissolved, pour in the orange juice and let it cool.
3. Slice and chop the rest of the orange. Toss it in a bowl with the apples, blueberries, and grapes.
4. Add the tea into the mixture to steep several minutes before serving.

Healthy Chocolate Granola
Time Required: 45-50 minutes
Servings: 8
Nutritional Calories: 193

Ingredients Needed:

- Cacao powder (.25 cup)
- Vanilla extract (.5 tsp.)
- Maple syrup (.25 cup)
- Melted coconut oil (2 tbsp.)
- Salt (1/8 tsp.)
- Coconut flakes (.25 cup - unsweetened)
- Gluten-free rolled oats (2 cups)
- Chia seeds (2 tbsp.)
- Unsweetened dark chocolate (2 tbsp.)

Method for Preparation:

1. Finely chop the chocolate.
2. Prepare a baking tray using a layer of parchment baking paper.

3. Warm the oven to reach 300° F/149° C.
4. Combine the syrup, cacao, oil, vanilla, and salt in a saucepan. Use the medium- temperature setting and simmer it for two to three minutes, stirring constantly.
5. Transfer it to the countertop to cool.
6. Toss the chia seeds, coconut, and oats in a large mixing container. Fold in the rest of the fixings and dump it onto the baking tray.
7. Set the timer for 35 minutes. Remove the pan and let it cool for about one hour. Add the chocolate chunks and stir well. Serve right away.

Sirt Muesli

Time Required: 30-35 minutes
Servings: 2
Nutritional Calories: 334

Ingredients Needed:

- Buckwheat drops (20g/.75 oz.)
- Buckwheat puffs (3/8 oz./10g)
- Dried coconut/coconut drops (.5 oz./15g)
- Medjool dates - hollowed and smashed - (1.5 oz./40g)
- Chopped pecans (.5 oz/15g)
- Cocoa nibs (3/8 oz./10g)
- Hulled & chopped strawberries (3.5 oz./100g)
- Plain Greek yogurt/Coconut yogurt/soya (3.5 oz/100g)

Method for Preparation:

1. Chop the pecans. Remove the hulls and chop the berries.
2. Combine each of the fixings.
3. Lastly, add the yogurt and berries right before it's served.

Vegan Banana Buckwheat Pancakes

Time Required: 20 minutes
Servings: 2 @ 3 pancakes each serving
Nutritional Calories: 107

Ingredients Needed:

- Buckwheat flour/ground groats (.5 cup)
- Bananas (2 whole/.75 of a cup - mashed)
- Olive/Coconut oil (2 tbsp.)
- Water (2 tbsp.)

- Vinegar - Apple cider (2 tsp.)
- Baking soda (.5 tsp.)
- Vanilla extract (1 tsp.)
- Cinnamon (1 tsp.)

Method for Preparation:

1. Set the oven temperature at 350° Fahrenheit/177 °Celsius to bake the pancakes.
2. Grind the buckwheat flour by pouring raw buckwheat groats into a coffee grinder. Grind to reach a fine flour-like texture (30 sec.) Measure the flour after grinding.
3. Mash the bananas and mix in with the oil, cinnamon, flour, water, baking soda, vanilla, and vinegar. Mix well - slightly thicker than traditional pancake batter.
4. Scoop the batter and make six mounds on a large parchment paper-lined baking tray.
5. Spread the pancakes out and bake until the centers are firm (15 min.) in the preheated oven.
6. You can also fry them in a skillet if desired. Prepare a skillet using the medium temperature setting. Dump a scant ¼ of a cup of batter into the pan. Let the top bubble (4-5 min.). Flip and cook on the other side.
7. Enjoy them hot with a serving of syrup and freshly prepared fruit.

Chapter 8: Sirtfood Poultry or Fish Option

Chicken Skewers With Satay Sauce
Time Required: 25-30 minutes
Servings: 1
Nutritional Calories: 974

Ingredients Needed:

- Chicken breast (150g)
- Olive oil (.5 tsp.)
- Buckwheat (50g)
- Ground turmeric (1 tsp.)
- Kale (30g)
- Celery (30g)
- Red onion (20g)
- Garlic clove (1)
- Olive oil (1 tsp.)
- Ground turmeric (1 tsp.)
- Curry powder (1 tsp.)
- Chicken stock (50 ml)
- Coconut milk (150 ml)
- Walnut butter or peanut butter (1 tbsp.)
- Coriander (1 tbsp.)
- To Garnish: Chopped walnut halves (4)

Method for Preparation:

1. Cut the chicken into chunks and mix it with turmeric and oil. Set aside to marinate (½ to one hour).
2. Remove the stalks and slice the kale and celery. Dice the onion, garlic, and coriander. Cook the buckwheat (per package guidelines), adding the kale and celery for the last five to seven minutes of the cooking time. Drain it in a colander.
3. Heat the grill on a high setting.
4. Cook the garlic and onion in oil until softened (2-3 min.). Stir in the spices and simmer for another minute.
5. Pour in the milk and stock. Wait for it to boil. Add the walnut butter and stir thoroughly. Lower the temperature setting and simmer the sauce for eight to ten minutes or until creamy.
6. As the sauce is simmering, thread the chicken on to the skewers, place them under the hot grill for ten minutes, and turn them after five minutes.
7. Stir in the coriander and pour it over the skewers. Scatter it using the chopped walnuts.

Vietnamese Turmeric Fish With Herbs & Mango Sauce

Total Time: 45-50 minutes/Marinate 1 hour to overnight
Servings Provided: 4
Calories: 345

Ingredients Needed:

- Fresh cod - boneless & skinless (1.25 lb.)
- Coconut oil (2 tbsp. to fry in a pan + more as needed)
- Sea salt (1 pinch)

Fish Marinate:

- Sea salt (1 tsp.)
- Turmeric powder (1 tbsp.)
- Chinese cooking wine or Dry sherry (1 tbsp.)
- Ginger - minced (2 tsp.)
- Olive oil (2 tbsp.)

Infused Oil:

- Fresh dill (2 cups)
- Scallions (2 cups/long thin strips)
- Sea salt (1 pinch/to your liking)

Mango Dipping Sauce:

- Ripe mango (1 medium)

- Garlic clove (1)
- Rice vinegar (2 tbsp.)
- Juice of ½ lime
- Dry red chili pepper - to serve (1 tsp.)

Toppings - As Desired:

- Lime juice
- Fresh cilantro
- Nuts (cashew/pine nuts)

Method for Preparation:

1. Prepare the fish. Cut it into a two-inch piece wide by ½ inch thick.
2. Marinate the fish as desired.
3. Toss each of the fixings under "*Mango Dipping Sauce*" into a food processor and pulse to reach the desired consistency.
4. Warm two tablespoons of oil in a big skillet using the high-temperature setting. Once it's hot, add the marinated fish and sprinkle them with salt. Cook them in two or more batches if needed.
5. Lower the heat to med-high once the fish start to sizzle.
6. Do *not* turn or move the fish until they are done on the first side (5 min.). Add more oil to the fish pan if necessary.
7. Carefully turn the fish and cook until they are done. Place them onto a large platter for now.
8. Use the remainder of the oil to make scallion-dill infused oil. Warm a skillet using the medium-high heat setting. Toss in two cups of scallions, and two cups of dill.
9. Extinguish the heat. Gently toss just until the scallions and dill have wilted (15 seconds). Season your meal with a dash of sea salt.
10. Pour the infused oil, scallion, and dill, and over the fish.
11. Serve the dish with the lime, nuts, fresh cilantro, and mango dipping sauce.

Chapter 9: Sirtfood Soup Options

Broccoli & Courgette Soup
Time Required: 20-25 minutes
Servings: 2
Nutritional Calories: 178

Ingredients Needed:

- Coconut oil (2 tbsp.)
- Red onion (1)
- Garlic (2 cloves)
- Broccoli (300g/10.5 oz.)
- Zucchini (1)
- Vegetable broth (24 fl. oz./750ml)

Method for Preparation:

1. Finely chop the garlic and onion, slice the zucchini, and cut the broccoli into florets.
2. Melt the oil in a soup pot. Sauté the garlic and onion. Fold in the zucchini to cook for a few minutes. Toss in the broccoli.
3. Pour in the broth and simmer the mixture for about five minutes.
4. Puree the soup with a hand blender. Garnish with pepper and salt as desired

Broccoli & Kale Green Soup
Time Required: 35-40 minutes
Servings: 2
Nutritional Calories: 182

Ingredients Needed:
- Stock (500 ml/2.1 cups)
- Sunflower oil (1 tbsp.)
- Cloves of garlic (2)
- Ginger (1-inch knob)
- Ground coriander (.5 tsp.)
- Fresh turmeric (1-inch piece/3cm)
- Pink Himalayan salt (1 pinch)
- Courgettes/cucumbers (200g)
- Broccoli (85g)
- Kale (100g)
- Lime (1 - zested & juiced)
- Parsley (small pack/as desired)

Method for Preparation:
1. Prepare the stock by mixing one tablespoon of bouillon powder and boiling water into a jug. Peel and grate the turmeric, and slice the ginger. Roughly chop the parsley.
2. Warm a deep skillet to warm the oil. Mince and toss in the ginger, garlic, turmeric, coriander, and salt. Sauté the mixture using the medium temperature setting for two minutes. Measure and add three tablespoons of water.
3. Roughly slice and add the courgettes, mixing well to coat the slices in all the spices and continue cooking for about three minutes.
4. Add 400ml stock and simmer them for about three minutes.
5. Toss in the kale, broccoli, and lime juice with the remainder of the stock.
6. Simmer the soup for another three to four minutes until all the veggies are softened.
7. Transfer the pan to the countertop and add the chopped parsley.
8. Toss all of the fixings into a blender and mix using the high-speed setting until the soup is creamy smooth.
9. Garnish the soup with lime zest and parsley to serve.

Lentil & Greens Soup
Time Required: 1 hour 10 minutes
Servings: 6
Nutritional Calories: 174

Ingredients Needed:

- Olive oil (1 tbsp.)
- Celery (2 stalks)
- Carrots (2)
- Yellow onion (1 medium)
- Cloves of garlic (3)
- Ground cumin (1.5 tsp.)
- Ground turmeric (1 tsp.)
- Red pepper flakes (.25 tsp.)
- Diced tomatoes (14.5 oz. can)
- Lentils (1 cup)
- Water (5.5 cups)
- Fresh mustard greens (2 cups)
- Lemon juice - freshly squeezed (2 tbsp.)
- Black pepper & salt (to your liking)

Method for Preparation:

1. Peel and chop the carrots and onion. Rinse the lentils.
2. Chop the celery and greens, and mince the garlic.
3. Warm the oil in a skillet using the medium temperature setting.
4. Sauté the onions, celery, and carrots for five to six minutes.
5. Toss in the garlic and spices. Simmer for about 60 seconds.
6. Dump in the tomatoes and simmer for two to three minutes.
7. Pour in the water and lentils. Wait for it to boil.
8. Adjust the temperature setting to low. Simmer with the lid on the pot for about 35 minutes.
9. Fold in the greens and simmer for about five more minutes.
10. At that point, add the juice, salt, and pepper.
11. Stir well and serve.

Shiitake Mushroom & Tofu Soup
Time Required: 30-35 minutes
Servings: 4
Nutritional Calories: 99

Ingredients Needed:

- Dried Wakame/seaweed (3/8 oz./10g)
- Vegetable stock (32 fl. oz./1 liter)
- Shiitake mushrooms (7 oz./200g)
- Firm tofu (14 oz./400g)
- Green onion (2)
- Bird's eye chili (1)

Method for Preparation:

1. Slice the mushrooms and dice the chili and tofu. Trim the onion and diagonally chop it.
2. Soak the Wakame in water for 10-15 minutes and drain it.
3. Prepare a medium saucepan with the vegetable stock. Wait for it to boil. Toss the mushrooms into the pan and simmer for two to three minutes.
4. Prepare the miso paste with three to four tablespoons of the vegetable stock until the miso is dissolved.
5. Pour the stock back into the pan, add the tofu, green onions, wakame, and chili. Stir and serve right away for the best results.

Chapter 10: Sirtfood Side Dish/Snack Options

Braised Puy Lentils
Time Required: 40-50 minutes
Servings: 1
Nutritional Calories: 521

Ingredients Needed:

- Cherry tomatoes (8)
- Olive oil (2 tsp.)
- Red onion (40g)
- Garlic clove (1)
- Celery (40g)
- Carrots (40g)
- Paprika (1 tsp.)
- Thyme - dry or fresh (1 tsp.)
- Puy lentils (75g)
- Vegetable stock (220 ml)
- Kale (50g)
- Parsley (1 tbsp.)
- Rocket (20g)

Method for Preparation:

1. Warm the oven to 248° Fahrenheit/120°Celsius/gas @ ½.
2. Slice the tomatoes into halves and toss them into a small roasting tin

and roast in the oven for 35 to 45 minutes.

3. Warm the oil in a saucepan using the low-med temperature setting.
4. Thinly slice the onion, celery, and peeled carrots. Mince the garlic and add the veggies into the pan to sauté them for one to two minutes until softened. Stir in the thyme and paprika. Sauté for one more minute.
5. Rinse the lentils in a fine-meshed sieve and add them to the pan with the stock. Wait for it to boil, and lower the heat. Simmer gently for 20 minutes with a lid on the pan.
6. Stir the components every seven minutes or so, adding a little water if the level drops too much.
7. Roughly chop and fold in the kale and cook for another ten minutes.
8. When the lentils are cooked, stir in the parsley and roasted tomatoes.
9. Serve with the rocket drizzled with the remaining teaspoon of olive oil.

Braised Pine Nuts & Leeks

Time Required: 15-20 minutes
Servings: 4
Nutritional Calories: 115

Ingredients Needed:

- Ghee (0.7 oz./20g)
- Olive oil (2 tsp.)
- Leek (2 pieces)
- Vegetable broth (.75 cup/5 fl. oz./150 ml)
- Fresh parsley (1 tbsp.)
- Roasted pine nuts (1 tbsp.)
- Fresh oregano (1 tbsp.)

Method for Preparation:

1. Cut the leek into thin rings and finely chop the herbs. Roast the pine nuts using the medium temperature setting in a dry frying pan. Set them aside.
2. Melt the ghee with the olive oil in the skillet.
3. Cook the leeks while continually stirring them for about five minutes until golden brown.
4. Add the vegetable broth and simmer for another ten minutes until the leek is softened.
5. Stir in the herbs and sprinkle the pine nuts over the dish just before serving.

Carrots & Kale
Time Required: 30-35 minutes
Servings: 4
Nutritional Calories: 166

Ingredients Needed:

- Olive oil (2 tbsp.)
- Small onion (1)
- Garlic cloves (3)
- Fresh kale (1 lb.)
- Carrots (.5 lb.)
- Raw honey (1 tbsp.)
- Juice (1 tbsp. / 1 lemon)
- Black pepper and salt (as desired)

Method for Preparation:

1. Chop the onion. Mince the garlic. Peel and shred the carrots. Lastly, remove the tough ribs from the kale and chop it to bits.
2. Heat a large wok using the medium temperature setting and add the oil.
3. Toss in the onion and sauté them for four to five minutes.
4. Stir in the garlic and sauté it for about 60 seconds.
5. Toss in the kale and sauté it for three to four minutes.
6. Add in the honey, lemon juice, carrots, black pepper, and salt.
7. Simmer for about four to five minutes and serve.

Fried Cauliflower Rice
Time Required: 55 minutes
Servings: 2
Nutritional Calories: 230

Ingredients Needed:

- Cauliflower (1 head)
- Coconut oil (2 tbsp.)
- Red onion (1)
- Garlic (4 cloves)
- Vegetable broth (2 fl. oz./60 ml.)
- Fresh ginger (1.5 cm/0.6-inch piece)
- Carrot (half of 1)
- Red bell pepper (half of 1)

- Chili flakes (1 tsp.)
- Lemon juice (half of 1 lemon)
- Pumpkin seeds (2 tbsp.)
- Fresh coriander (2 tbsp.)

Method for Preparation:
1. Use a food processor to 'rice' the cauliflower. Finely chop the ginger, garlic, and onion. Slice the carrot into thin matchsticks, finely chop the herbs and dice the bell pepper.
2. Melt the oil in a skillet, adding half of the garlic and onion. Sauté until the onion is translucent. Toss in salt and the rice.
3. Mix in the broth and stir until the rice is tender. When ready, remove it from the pan in a mixing container.
4. Melt the remainder of the oil in the pan and toss in the rest of the veggies. Sauté them until they are tender. Toss in everything and heat.
5. Spritz with the juice and garnish with the seeds and coriander to serve.

Italian Kale - Gluten-Free - Vegetarian
Time Required: 10-15 minutes
Servings: 8
Nutritional Calories: 50

Ingredients Needed:
- Olive oil (3 tbsp.)
- Garlic (3 cloves)
- Wine vinegar (3 tbsp. - red)
- Kale (300g)

Method for Preparation:
1. Warm the oil in a large skillet with a lid. Mince and sauté the garlic. Mix in the vinegar with a splash of water.
2. Toss the kale into the pan, cover with a lid, and wilt in the steam for four to five minutes, adding a splash more water if needed.
3. After it's wilted, sprinkle it with a bit of sea salt, and serve.

Kale & Pine Nuts
Time Required: 20-25 minutes
Servings: 4

Nutritional Calories: 146

Ingredients Needed:

- Olive oil (1 tbsp.)
- Garlic (2 cloves)
- Fresh kale (1.5 lb.)
- Water (.25 cup)
- Red wine vinegar (3 tsp.)
- Pine nuts (2 tbsp.)
- Black pepper and salt (as desired)

Method for Preparation:

1. Remove the tough ribs from the kale and chop it. Mince the garlic.
2. Warm the oil in a wok using the medium temperature setting.
3. Toss in and sauté the garlic for one minute. Toss in the kale and sauté them for three to four minutes.
4. Pour in the water, salt, pepper, and vinegar. Simmer for four to five minutes.
5. Transfer it from the heat and mix in the pine nuts.
6. Serve and enjoy them right away for the best flavor results.

Kale With Lemon Tahini Dressing

Time Required: 10 minutes
Servings: 2
Nutritional Calories: 274

Ingredients Needed:

- Water (50ml)
- Juice (3 tbsp./1 lemon)
- Tahini (50g)
- Garlic (1 clove)
- Olive oil (1 tbsp.)
- Kale (200g)

Method for Preparation:

1. Mince the garlic and juice the lemon.
2. Prepare the dressing. Whisk the garlic, lemon juice, tahini, and cold

water in a small mixing container. Season the dressing to your liking.

3. Warm the oil in a large skillet and stir-fry the kale for three minutes.
4. Add half of the dressing to the pan and continue to cook for another 30 seconds. Dump the kale into a serving bowl and drizzle it using the rest of the dressing.

Chapter 11: Sirtfood Salad Options

Arugula Salad In A Jar - Carrots - Buckwheat & Tomatoes
Time Required: 30-35 minutes
Servings: 2
Nutritional Calories: 293

Ingredients Needed:

- Sunflower seeds (.5 cup)
- Carrots (.5 cup)
- Shredded cabbage (.5 cup)
- Tomatoes (.5 cup)
- Cooked buckwheat (1 cup) mixed with chia seeds (1 tbsp.)
- Arugula (1 cup)

The Dressing:

- Juice (1 lemon/1 tbsp.)
- Olive oil (1 tbsp.)
- Sea salt (1 pinch)

Method for Preparation:

1. Prepare the jar:
   - Pour in the dressing
   - Cabbage

- Sunflower seeds
- Carrots
- Buckwheat
- Tomatoes
- Arugula

2. It's perfect for a grab-and-go option!

Kale - Raspberry Salad
Time Required: 15 minutes
Servings: 2
Nutritional Calories: 228

Ingredients Needed:

- Fresh baby kale (3 cups)
- Chopped walnuts (.25 cup)
- Fresh raspberries (.5 cup)

The Dressing:

- Olive oil (1 tbsp.)
- Pure maple syrup (.5 tsp.)
- Apple cider vinegar (1 tbsp.)
- Salt and black pepper (as desired)

Method for Preparation:

1. Toss each of the salad fixings into two salad bowls.
2. Combine the dressing in another container. Shake the mixture thoroughly until mixed.
3. Add the dressing to the salad and serve.

Orange Rocket Salad
Time Required: 10 minutes
Servings: 4
Nutritional Calories: 233

Ingredients Needed:

- Oranges (3 large)
- Beets (2)
- Fresh rocket (6 cups)
- Walnuts (.25 cup)
- Olive oil (3 tbsp.)
- Salt (1 pinch)

Method for Preparation:

1. Peel and remove the seeds from the oranges. Trim the beets, peel, and slice. Chop the walnuts and rinse the rocket. Toss it all into a salad mixing bowl.
2. Serve right away for the best results.

Watercress - Strawberry - Tomato Salad With Pink Pepper & Honey Dressing

Time Required: 10-15 minutes
Servings: 4
Nutritional Calories: 128
Ingredients Needed:

- Watercress (100g)
- Strawberries (300g)
- Mixed tomatoes (250g)

The Dressing:

- Strawberries (2/40g/chopped)
- Honey (.5 tbsp.)
- Lemon (half of 1 - juiced)
- Juice (half of 1 lemon)
- Pink peppercorns (1 tbsp.)
- Olive oil (3 tbsp.)

Method for Preparation:

1. Discard the watercress stalks. Juice the lemon.
2. Prepare the dressing. Toast the peppercorns in a dry skillet until fragrant (1-2 min.). Break the skins using a pestle and mortar with a pinch of salt. Add two strawberries and mash them to a paste.
3. Mix in the honey and lemon juice. Pour the dressing into a large bowl and whisk in the oil. Adjust the seasoning as desired.
4. Assemble the salad. Cut the strawberries into quarters/wedges, and roughly chop the tomatoes. Mix with the watercress in the bowl.
5. Divide the salad between four plates and serve any dressing left in a bowl.

Waldorf Salad

Time Required: 10-15 minutes
Servings: 2
Nutritional Calories: 275

Ingredients Needed:

- Celery (200g)

- Apple (100g)
- Walnuts (50g)
- Red onion (1 small)
- Chicory (1 head)
- Flat parsley (10g)
- Capers (1 tbsp.)
- Lovage or celery leaves (10g)

The Dressing:

- Extra virgin olive oil (1 tbsp.)
- Balsamic vinegar (1 tsp.)
- Dijon mustard (1 tsp.)
- Juice of ½ lemon

Method for Preparation:

1. Roughly chop the apple, lovage, celery, onion, and walnuts. Chop the parsley and chicory.
2. Combine the lovage, capers, parsley, celery, walnuts, onion, and apple in a salad bowl.
3. Whisk the dressing components (lemon juice, mustard, vinegar, and oil).
4. Drizzle the dressing over the delicious salad and serve!

Chapter 12: Sirtfood Snacks

Delicious Smoothies

Berry Smoothie
Time Required: 5 minutes
Servings: 1
Nutritional Calories: 195

Ingredients Needed:
- Courgette (half of 1 medium)
- Mixed berries (1 cup - frozen)
- Avocado (half of 1)
- Vegan Berry Protein Powder (1 heaping tbsp.)
- Unsweetened dairy-free milk (as needed)

Method for Preparation:
1. Peel and slice the courgette/cucumber. Roughly chop the avocado.
2. Add all of the ingredients into a blender and mix.
3. Serve in a frosty mug.

Green Tea Smoothies
Time Required: 3-6 minutes
Servings: 2
Nutritional Calories: 183

Ingredients Needed:
- Ripe bananas (2)

- Milk (250 ml)
- Vanilla bean paste - not extract (.5 tsp.) or (a small scrape of the seeds from a vanilla pod)
- Matcha green tea powder (2 tsp.)
- Ice (6 cubes)
- Honey (2 tsp.)

Method for Preparation:
1. Measure and add all of the components into a blender.
2. Mix well and serve them in two chilled glasses.

Other Treats

Apricot Granola
Time Required: 25-30 minutes
Servings: 8
Nutritional Calories: 177

Ingredients Needed:
- Oats (200g)
- Chia Seeds (20g)
- Flaked almonds (20g)
- Flaxseeds (20g)
- Coconut oil (10g)
- Mild olive oil (30ml)
- Malt extract (40g)
- Dried apricots (40g)

Method for Preparation:
1. Warm the oven to 160° Celsius/325° Fahrenheit. Prepare a large baking tray using a layer of parchment baking paper.
2. Combine the oats, chia, flaxseeds, and almonds in a mixing container.
3. Combine the oils and malt extract in a small saucepan until warm, combined, and pourable.
4. Pour the liquids into the oat mix and stir gently until evenly coated.
5. Tip the mix on to the baking sheet and untidily spread around.
6. Bake for 20 minutes.
7. Let cool in the tray. Chop the apricots and mix them into the granola.
8. Keep in an airtight container.

Matcha Iced Chocolate Cupcakes
Time Required: 35 minutes
Servings: 12
Nutritional Calories: 234

Ingredients Needed:

- Caster sugar (200g)
- Self-rising flour (150g)
- Salt (.5 tsp.)
- Cocoa (60g)
- Fine espresso coffee (.5 tsp.)
- Milk (120ml)
- Vanilla extract (.5 tsp.)
- Boiling water (120ml)
- Vegetable oil (50ml)
- Egg (1)

The Icing:

- Icing sugar (50g)
- Unchilled butter (50g)
- Matcha green tea powder (1 tbsp.)
- Soft cream cheese (50g)
- Vanilla bean paste (.5 tsp.)

Method for Preparation:

1. Warm the oven to 356° Fahrenheit/180° Celsius/160° Celsius fan. Line a cupcake tin with paper/silicone cake cases.
2. Whisk the flour, cocoa, sugar, espresso powder, and salt in a large mixing bowl.
3. Stir in the milk, vegetable oil, vanilla extract, and egg to the dry components. Use an electric mixer to combine until fully incorporated.
4. Slowly pour in the boiling water. Mix using the low-speed setting until the mixture is thoroughly combined.
5. Continue using the high-speed setting to mix for another minute. The batter should be more liquidy than regular cake batter.
6. Spoon the batter between each of the molds (¾ full). Bake them until the mixture bounces back when tapped (15-18 min.).
7. Completely cool them before decorating.
8. Cream the butter and icing sugar until it's pale and smooth.
9. Add in the vanilla and matcha powder.
10. Lastly, add the cream cheese and mix until it's creamy. Pipe or spread over the cupcakes to serve.

Walnut-Date Cinnamon Bites
Time Required: 5 minutes
Servings: 1
Nutritional Calories: 168

Ingredients Needed:

- Walnut halves (3)
- Medjool dates (3 pitted)
- Ground cinnamon (as desired)

Method for Preparation:

1. Slice each half of the walnuts into three slices.
2. Add a nut on top of each date.
3. Serve with a dusting of cinnamon.

Conclusion

I hope you have and will enjoy each segment of the Sirtfood Diet Cookbook. I hope it was informative and provided you with all of the tools you need to achieve your goals while on the diet.

The next step is to gather your shopping list and head to the market for the goodies to prepare your first days of the plan using the dieting techniques used in your new cookbook.

Let's briefly highlight the benefits you will acquire using the Sirtfood Diet.

- Activate the same skinny genes in your body that fasting triggers.
- Effectively lose weight and improve your disease resistance.
- The plan can provide you with incredible energy and glowing health.
- Lose Fat While Eating Delicious Food!
- Retain your muscle mass.
- You should have improved memory function.
- You should acquire more control of your blood sugar levels.
- Reduced hunger or cravings is a plus. You won't be hungry while on the Sirtfood Diet!

Stay determined as you begin your new diet plan. You will probably have a few side effects when you begin your new plan with just the juices as your baseline for the first week, but you will move past that and enjoy full menus with more than you usually eat and still drop the pounds.

No diet is easy, but you can be successful by taking the extra time and energy to prepare a plan that will work for you. You have a ton of new ways to lose weight, as outlined in your 28-day meal plan. However, the road to success will be one you will be glad you took! Try it short-term. If you like how it makes you feel at the end of the phases up to 21 days, try it again for another round. While you are taking a pause, maybe you could try some of the other recipes - not on the prepared meal plan.

Finally, if you found this cookbook useful in any way, a review on Amazon is always appreciated!

Lightning Source UK Ltd.
Milton Keynes UK
UKHW020643240521
384271UK00011B/771